CARRYING A
LITTLE EXTRA

CARRYING A LITTLE EXTRA

A GUIDE TO HEALTHY PREGNANCY FOR THE PLUS–SIZE WOMAN

PAULA BERNSTEIN, PH.D., M.D.,

MARLENE CLARK, R.D.,

AND NETTY LEVINE, M.S., R.D.

BERKLEY BOOKS, NEW YORK

B

A Berkley Book
Published by The Berkley Publishing Group
A division of Penguin Putnam Inc.
375 Hudson Street
New York, New York 10014

Every effort has been made to ensure that the information contained in this book
is complete and accurate. However, neither the publisher nor the authors are
engaged in rendering professional advice or services to the individual reader.
The ideas, procedures, and suggestions contained in this book are not intended
as a substitute for consulting with your physician. All matters regarding your
health require medical supervision. Neither the authors nor the publisher shall be
liable or responsible for any loss, injury or damage allegedly arising from any
information or suggestion in this book. The opinions expressed in this book
represent the personal views of the authors and not of the publisher.

PRINTING HISTORY
Berkley trade paperback edition / February 2003

Library of Congress Cataloging-in-Publication Data

Bernstein, Paula.
Carrying a little extra : a guide to healthy pregnancy for the plus-size woman /
Paula Bernstein, Marlene Clark, and Netty Levine.
p. cm.
Includes index.
ISBN 0-425-18834-5
1. Pregnancy. 2. Pregnancy—Complications. 3. Overweight women.
4. Women—Health and hygiene. I. Clark, Marlene, R.D. II. Levine, Netty.
III. Title.

RG556 .B454 2003
618.2—dc21
2002027808

PRINTED IN THE UNITED STATES OF AMERICA

10 9 8 7 6 5 4 3 2 1

Dedicated to the memory of our moms: Beverly Ostrov, Lilly Wachtenheim and Anna Kreisman; and in honor of another special mom, Haya Wachtenheim and the six children who made us moms: Danielle, Jessica, Jonathan, Lauren, Samantha, and Zachary.

CONTENTS

Part II
NUTRITIONAL CONSIDERATIONS FOR A
HEALTHY PREGNANCY

ACKNOWLEDGMENTS

Several people contributed their inspiration and expertise to making this book happen. We thank Angela Rinaldi, our literary agent, and Christine Zika, our hardworking editor at Penguin Putnam. Dr. Uri Bernstein gave us tireless computer assistance, and Jessica Levine Kupferberg donated witty contributions to our chapter titles. We thank Jeffrey A. Clark for his legal advice and our kids for putting up with us during the writing process. A special thanks to Jean Larkin, who was the inspiration for our group collaboration.

INTRODUCTION AND A PERSONAL NOTE

n times past, the general public, including physicians, regarded overweight as some kind of character disorder. The classic stereotype was the fat woman standing in front of an open refrigerator at midnight, shoveling in huge quantities of ice cream, doughnuts, and french fries. If only she exercised some willpower and self-control, the theory went, she could lose all that extra weight and be normal. Overweight individuals were perceived as lazy, sloppy, and emotionally defective.

Generations of women bought into this battering of their self-esteem and tried desperately to lose weight. Weight loss became a major industry in the United States. People have tried everything: Weight Watchers, Overeaters Anonymous, TOPS, Pritikin, the Atkins Diet, the Zone Diet, the 500-calorie protein-powder starvation diet, not to mention the enormous number of herbal supplements, diet pills, and miracle foods advertised to make over your body in two weeks' time.

In the meantime, medical researchers struggled to answer the question of why it appeared to be so difficult for people to sustain long-term weight loss. Anyone who has lost and gained the same twenty or thirty pounds a dozen times is familiar with the problem. Our understanding is still incomplete, but it has become increasingly clear that overweight is far more a question of genetics and metabolism than of willpower.

The evidence is also clear that excess weight confers excess risk on women during and after pregnancy and may be a trigger for the further development of obesity.

The purpose of this book is to optimize chances for a healthy pregnancy and delivery for women who struggle with their weight. It is not another diet book. Our goals are to provide women with accurate medical information about the increased risks of being overweight during pregnancy and to suggest sensible, achievable nutritional strategies before, during, and after pregnancy. We want to help mothers gain enough weight to deliver a healthy baby while avoiding the risks of excessive pounds.

This book is divided into two parts—obstetrical information and nutritional information. The first half discusses what current research tells us about overweight and explains how weight affects fertility. It reviews the medical evidence for increased risk during pregnancy, labor and delivery, and postpartum, and explains in simple terms the nature of the medical problems and how to manage them.

The second half of the book presents strategies for healthy eating. It explains the nutritional requirements of pregnancy and how they vary depending upon the woman's starting weight. Diet plans and menus are presented for use during pregnancy, for breast-feeding, and postpartum weight loss. The special requirements of women who become diabetic in the course of pregnancy will also be reviewed.

This book is a professional collaboration between two

skinny dietitians and one unabashedly overweight obstetrician. Between us we have close to seventy-five years of experience in helping women to have healthy pregnancies. It is our hope that this book will serve as a resource for women who are carrying a little extra, and who are motivated to make their pregnancies as healthy as possible.

Paula's Story

All of the women in my family, for generations, have been *zaftig*. That's Yiddish for "well endowed." No one, except my teenage daughter, who inherited all of my recessive thin genes, has ever worn a single-digit size. I distinctly recall going on my first diet at the age of five. The diet plan consisted of restricting myself to no more than one chocolate per day out of the large box of Schrafft's that my mother had placed so temptingly on the coffee table. Even at age five, I considered it unlikely that the baby fat, which looked so cute in my toddler photos, would magically disappear as I grew taller.

Junior high school, high school, and college were a roller coaster of yo-yo dieting. I was convinced that if only I could lose 20 or 30 pounds I would be beautiful, popular, and have boyfriends. As I look back at photos from that time in my life, I wonder what it was I could have been thinking. I had a 29-inch waist in high school and was mortified that it wasn't 24. Where did I get that idea? I'd love to have a 29-inch waist now, or for that matter anything I could identify as a waist.

After college in New York, I moved to California to go to graduate school at Caltech. Four years later, I graduated with a Ph.D., considerable knowledge about the arcane aspects of transition metal chemistry, and an extremely nice husband. I've forgotten most of the chemistry, but I did hang on to the husband.

During my years in graduate school and the early years of

my marriage, my weight stayed fairly stable. This was probably because, for the first time in my life, I was actually getting some exercise. In all honesty, my favorite form of workout is, and has always been, hiking from the sofa to the refrigerator, carrying a really good novel. I had, however, married a man whose concept of the perfect vacation was backpacking up a steep slope in the Sierras carrying 50 pounds of gear. As an ex–New Yorker, I'd never camped in my life, but I was in love. I learned to hike, backpack, river-raft, rock-climb, and rappel my way down cliffs.

During the next two years, I pursued postdoctoral fellowships and looked for academic jobs in chemistry. Unfortunately, academic jobs in general were exceptionally scarce at that time, and finally I decided to change careers and apply to medical school. The University of Miami had created a program that seemed tailor-made for me—a two-year curriculum for people who already had a Ph.D. in science.

I was accepted, and headed east for two years of frizzy hair, palmetto bugs, and the most intense academic work I'd ever experienced. After a stressful time of applying to medical schools, looking for jobs, and feeling completely uncertain about the future, my weight was at its all-time high.

I was determined that medicine would allow me to accomplish two goals: to maintain my autonomy and to do something constructive for other women. Obstetrics and gynecology fit my needs with the precision of a surgical glove. During my second year in medical school, I decided once again that I had to lose weight. With an extraordinary amount of willpower, I restricted myself to 1000 calories a day for an entire year, shedding 60 pounds in the process. When I started my internship, back in Los Angeles, I was at an all-time minimum weight, having no doubt driven my poor husband to distraction with my obsessive behavior over food.

It wasn't difficult to keep the weight off during most of residency. Being a resident is a physically exhausting process. Senior year, however, I bent over a patient to listen to her lungs and couldn't stand up again. I'd slipped a disk, winding up in the hospital in traction for ten days and in a back brace for six months thereafter. The pounds started to creep up again.

After residency I started my private practice. One of the perks of the job was getting to play with the babies I'd delivered, and after a while this reminded me that I was no spring chicken. I'd put off having children while I finished my Ph.D., my M.D., and my residency training. If I was planning to have any, now was the time.

Like many overweight women, my cycles were not always regular, and I was approaching forty. I started myself on the fertility drug Clomid, and started using an ovulation predictor kit. Much to my surprise, I did not get pregnant on the first try—or the second—or the third. In fact, it took a leisurely vacation (during which I forgot my ovulation predictor kit) to do the job. This convinced me that stress truly does affect fertility, and I often prescribe a vacation during ovulation time to my patients who seem to be having trouble conceiving.

At the time I became pregnant I was forty years old and probably about that many pounds overweight, but otherwise in good health. I wasn't diabetic or hypertensive. My main concerns for the pregnancy had to do with not straining my vulnerable back, and not gaining a huge amount of weight that I would have to struggle to lose.

The weight turned out not to be a problem. Some women have a huge appetite during pregnancy and will eat anything that isn't tied down. I found that the hormones of pregnancy made me practically anorexic. Although I wasn't actually nauseated, the sight of most of my favorite foods was completely unappealing, and I had to force myself to get down the things I knew my baby required for healthy development. During my first trimester, I lost nine pounds.

I had enlisted my associate as my obstetrician. I trusted her judgment more than anyone else's, and I knew she would keep me safe. She was also the only person I could think of who would let me get away without weighing myself during my obstetrical exams. I'd always considered my weight something of an embarrassment and a state secret. There was no way I was going to have it on my chart, in the file cabinet in Labor and Delivery, where the entire nursing and resident staff could read it. (I can't imagine why I thought they'd be interested!) We came to an agreement. I'd weigh myself, and tell her how many pounds I'd gained or lost since the prior visit. We got to plus-16 pounds before I delivered.

Things were progressing nicely until I got to twenty-six weeks. Then suddenly, we noticed that the baby was falling off the growth curve. Ultrasounds showed her to be in the tenth percentile for her gestational age, a diagnosis called IUGR (intrauterine growth retardation). IUGR can be a result of a number of factors, hypertension and stress being two of the most common. The usual remedy is bed rest, and I was sent home with orders to take it easy.

I am not someone who does well "taking it easy" and I didn't especially enjoy bed rest. I did manage to refinance the mortgage on my house and order the nursery furniture while I was in bed, but I was cranky. To tell the truth, my entire office staff threatened to resign if I ever got pregnant again.

We continued to follow the baby with ultrasounds, and she continued to grow, but only on the tenth percentile growth curve. In the meantime, my blood pressure began to rise and I started to spill protein in my urine. This answered the question of why the baby was IUGR. Early toxemia of pregnancy can certainly cut the blood flow to the placenta. At thirty-one weeks things began to deteriorate. The ultrasound showed that the right ventricle of my daughter's heart was beginning to dilate as a result of trying to pump blood back to a placenta with high resistance. In addition, she was falling off the growth curve. We had reached the point where she was clearly going to be better off outside the uterus than inside. It was time to deliver.

There comes a moment in every pregnancy when the mother realizes that the baby is actually going to have to come out. Even for someone who knew all the facts and who'd delivered hundreds of other women, it was a slightly terrifying realization.

I was admitted to the hospital and treated for forty-eight hours with steroids to mature the baby's lungs, and then taken to the operating room for a cesarean section. My daughter was breech, which made the decision to do a cesarean obvious, but I would not have wanted her subject to the stress of labor in any case. The surgery was performed by my partner, assisted by the husband of another dear friend, who was also there with her camera, my husband being too nervous to be trusted for photos. I'd selected my favorite anesthesiologist to administer the epidural and I was watching as they pulled out a 2-pound 11-ounce breech baby girl and handed her over to the neonatology staff.

My miniature daughter was a feisty little thing and had no problem breathing. She did, however, have to stay in the neonatal intensive care unit for the next seven weeks, until she gained enough weight to make it safe to take her home.

I had been under the illusion that the lack of appetite that had characterized my pregnancy would continue into the postpartum period. Unfortunately, this turned out not to be the case. As the placenta was removed from my uterus, I experienced an intense desire for pizza. I found it annoying that this wasn't on the clear liquid menu I was given the next day.

I found the experience of having a cesarean very easy and my recovery was rapid. The very next day I walked the halls, stopping to make rounds on two of my patients. On my tenth postoperative day, I delivered a baby and I was able to return to the office in two weeks. Being in the office all day made it easier to visit my baby in the NICU, and gave some relief to my partner, who had been juggling two practices for two months and was exhausted. I paid her back for that favor when she got pregnant.

Once we brought Danielle home from the hospital, I was much too busy being enchanted with my daughter to even think about my weight, which increased yet again. After a while I tried returning to my trusty 1000-calorie a day diet, on which I'd always managed to lose five pounds the first week and a pound a week thereafter. To my surprise, I discovered that things no longer worked that way with a forty-year-old metabolism. If I wanted to lose weight, I might actually have to exercise. One of my favorite patients, an exercise video guru, supplied me with all her exercise tapes and a set of weights. This resulted in my reclaiming my flabby abdominal muscles and building up my thighs. In a flood of enthusiasm I actually hired a personal trainer. (This is someone who lives in Los Angeles, has a perfect body, and charges money to torture you.) Things went well for some months, and I was actually in better physical shape than I'd been in years, until the day my trainer decided it would be fun to do step aerobics. I twisted my knee coming off the step, tore my medial meniscus, and landed in the hospital for arthroscopic surgery. I canceled the trainer.

One afternoon, when Danielle was about three, she and I and my husband were driving somewhere. Out of the blue, this little voice from the backseat said, "Mommy, are you fat?"

I hemmed and hawed for a minute or so and she asked the question again.

"Mommy, are you fat?"

"Yes, Danielle," I finally admitted. "I'm fat."

There was a pause.

"Mommy," she said, "when I grow up, can I be fat like you?"

I think that was the moment I had my epiphany. It was clear

to me that I had successfully managed to accomplish almost everything I'd ever wanted to do in my life. I'd finished a Ph.D. I'd gotten an M.D. in only two years. I had a wonderful husband, an adorable child, a large number of devoted friends, and a successful practice. I'd even managed to finish writing five novels in my spare time. (No, I haven't sold any of them yet, but that's my next project.)

The only thing I'd ever failed to do was lose weight and keep it off. Clearly this wasn't a question of ability and willpower. Anyone with the willpower to write five novels is not lacking in this department. Perhaps, I thought, it is simply not possible to triumph over one's genetics and metabolism. Furthermore, it occurred to me that being thin wasn't going to get me anything I didn't already have. It wasn't going to get me a nicer husband, a cuter child, better friends, or a more successful practice. The only thing it might get me was into a Giorgio Armani suit, and frankly, what with managed care and school tuition, I couldn't afford Armani. I decided to buy some beautiful new clothes and stop dieting.

That was twelve years ago. I haven't lost much, but I haven't gained anything either. I discovered that as long as I don't go overboard with eating, my body more or less maintains itself at a stable weight. I avoid fast food, try not to buy junk food, and concentrate on low-fat and nonfat products. We grill and eat lots of salads. If I'm not hungry, I don't bother eating.

As a physician, I've seen both ends of the weight spectrum. I'm very much aware of all the data demonstrating that significant obesity increases hypertension, diabetes, coronary artery disease, and mortality. I also see the teenagers and young Hollywood actresses who obsess over their weight and who are anorexic and bulimic.

I don't weigh my patients as part of their routine examinations unless they are pregnant. If a woman is overweight, she already knows it and doesn't need me to put her on the scale to demonstrate it. There is nothing more annoying than a sanctimonious physician (usually a thin one) lecturing on the subject of weight loss. If someone wants to discuss her weight and needs help, I try to do three things. First, I encourage realistic goals. Second, I encourage a degree of comfort and self-acceptance of body type and body weight. This is not easy in Los Angeles, where everyone feels inadequate if they don't look as if they just walked off the cover of *Vogue*. Finally, I send them to Netty and Marlene for nutritional guidance. I usually point out that there is no magic formula. If there were, I'd be a size eight.

A Word from Netty and Marlene

Writing the nutrition portion of this book couldn't be more appropriate for two best-friend dietitians who really bonded over pregnancy.

Netty's Story

When I became pregnant at age twenty-one, the weight-gain goal for all pregnant women was 24 pounds. Becoming pregnant unexpectedly, I had no time to read about what to eat before getting pregnant. Even if I had time, reading was impossible because I suffered from hyperemesis (nausea and vomiting in pregnancy). In the early hours of the morning, I was in the bathroom throwing up. I looked liked like Pippi Longstocking with broken blood vessels in my cheeks. My doctor told me to avoid fatty foods, but the only thing that worked for me was a greasy cold grilled-cheese sandwich. I lost 5 pounds in the first trimester with my daughter, Jessica, but ended up gaining 24 pounds by the end of the pregnancy. Twenty-nine years later, Jessica has given birth to my granddaughter, Kayla!

My second pregnancy was also unexpected. I guess I was not too smart in those days. This time, the only thing I could keep down was eight ounces of nonfat milk with one tablespoon of coffee ice cream floating on top. Once again, I lost five pounds during the first trimester. As soon as I felt better, I went back to my well-balanced diet. Jonathan, who is soon to be a doctor, was the result.

Things were different with Zachary, my number three. This pregnancy was my only planned pregnancy. I was sicker than ever. That is when Marlene and I became best friends—twenty-one years ago. She had returned from maternity leave only to find me vomiting in her trash can. Marlene knew. She knew that she would be covering for me in less than nine months. Zac is soon to be a college senior.

Marlene's Story

My pregnancies were more eventful than Netty's but less eventful than Paula's. Both of my daughters, Lauren and Samantha, were born one month early. I had gained over 30 pounds with each and they each weighed about 5½ pounds but were healthy little girls. In the first few months of my pregnancies, I, too, had morning sickness and was spending the mornings over the trash can in my office. Was this a dietitian thing? I remember a few weeks in particular when I resorted to all "white" foods. As long as the food didn't have color, it didn't bother me. Vanilla milk shakes, turkey sandwiches on white bread, and mashed potatoes were my comfort foods. After that phase, I ate by "trial and error." I worried about the effect of the "morning, noon, and night" sickness, but since my mom had experienced the same problems during her three pregnancies, she reassured me that everything would be fine. As time marched on, I started to feel better and I could eat more food. My two daughters are now twenty-one and eighteen. They are about to graduate from college and high school. We all try to eat a healthy diet and exercise regularly. They know I don't believe in dieting because they've heard me say a million times, "If you eat when you're hungry and stop when you're full, you won't need a diet." They've learned to pay attention to internal cues about hunger instead of external cues such as the clock. I've also taught them to recognize emotional eating such as eating when they are stressed or bored. These suggestions have worked well for my family but may not work for other families, whose genetic makeup is entirely different.

Pregnancy is a time where the issues of weight gain loom large. We've reviewed the medical literature on this subject extensively, and there is no question that overweight women are at higher risk for a number of complications of pregnancy, delivery, and the postpartum period. This doesn't mean that every plus-sized woman will have a complication, but it does mean that careful preconceptual planning and good prenatal care are essential. The more you know, the more actively you can participate in optimizing health for yourself and your baby. It is in this spirit that the three of us have written *Carrying a Little Extra*.

CARRYING A LITTLE EXTRA

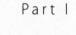

Part I

THE EFFECTS OF OVERWEIGHT AND OBESITY ON FERTILITY AND PREGNANCY

Chapter One

Why We Weigh What We Weigh

Defining Overweight and Obesity

Health professionals have long known that overweight is a contributing factor to many different diseases and medical complications. Furthermore, the percentage of adults in the United States who are overweight or obese has been gradually increasing, making obesity a major health problem.

In order to define overweight and obesity in a consistent manner, physicians use a term called the *BMI* or *body mass index*. The BMI relates weight to height and can be easily calculated.

BMI = body weight in kilograms ÷ (height in meters)^2

The easiest way to determine your BMI is to consult the table at the end of this chapter.

The term *overweight* refers to a BMI between 25 and 29.9.

Obesity is defined as a BMI over 30.[1] Researchers are not consistent in their definition of *morbid obesity*. Some use a BMI of over 33, some use over 40.

Several government agencies have studied the prevalence of obesity in the United States. One study has demonstrated that obesity has increased from 12 percent of the adult population in 1991 to 17.9 percent in 1998.[2, 3] Another, done in 1999, suggests that 61 percent of adults in our country are either overweight or obese.[4]

Despite the magnitude of the problem, the solution continues to elude us. Many years of research have made it clear that the causes of obesity are multiple and complex, and that most strategies that have been employed to lose weight permanently have failed. In the following chapter we will summarize some of the most recent research into the factors that regulate body weight and look at some of the more promising approaches to weight loss.

The Role of Genetics

New methods of genetic research and the unraveling of the human genome promise major leaps in our understanding and treatment of obesity. *It is now clear, from both animal and human studies, that the susceptibility to obesity is controlled by our genes.*[5]

Most of our information on the genetics of obesity comes from studies on animal models. This is because it is much easier to control mice than men. The experimenter can control the amount and nutritional content of the diet as well as the amount of exercise. A very important fact that we have learned from animal models is that there are many different genes that control obesity, scattered over many different chromosomes. There is no one, dominant "obesity gene" that determines weight.

This is quite different from the simplified genetics, first discovered by Mendel, that many of us learned in school.

What kind of evidence do we have that genetics play a major role in human obesity? Studies involving over 100,000 people examined relationships between identical twins, fraternal twins, parents and their natural children, and parents and their adoptive children.[6] The largest similarity in BMI occurred in identical twins, with almost no correlation between parents and their adopted children. The sum of all of these studies examined together suggests that between 50 percent and 90 percent of the time, BMI is dependent upon genetic inheritance.

Can we conclude anything about human beings from research done on mice? Actually, we can learn an enormous amount from animal models. The genetic structure of most mammals is remarkably similar. Only a very small fraction of our DNA distinguishes us from the ape, or from the laboratory rat. Thus, if a gene is identified in a mouse, we have a good idea of where to look for a similar gene in humans. At present, a "human obesity gene map"[7] has been established that contains more than forty genes and fifteen chromosomal regions in which there is a possible relationship to human overweight.

It is not enough merely to locate a gene. We must understand in detail what that particular gene does. Each individual gene is a code for a specific protein that becomes part of a more complex biochemical mechanism in the body. The protein may be involved in inducing or shutting off appetite. It may help conserve or use energy. It may be involved in the pathways that burn or store fat. As we begin to unravel the pathways for each gene, we may be able to identify places where we can block or enhance the action of the protein. This may lead to new therapeutic avenues for the treatment of obesity.

The Role of Environment

Despite the fact that genetics determine how susceptible an individual is to becoming obese, environment clearly plays a role as well. Obesity is a disease of affluent, first-world countries. For most of human history, people have spent their time doing hard physical labor and worrying about obtaining enough food. Thus we have evolved into a species that is very efficient at obtaining energy and that stores fat in order to survive times of potential starvation.[8] In primitive cultures, obesity was a sign of wealth. Being fat meant that you had more than enough to eat, and had servants to do your hard physical work. In an affluent culture, such as exists today in the United States, high-fat food is as close as the nearest McDonald's. No one is starving, and people spend most of their time sitting in front of their computers or TV screens. The days of chopping wood or hunting for dinner are long gone. Thus, *genes that may confer a survival advantage in cultures where food is scarce and physical activity is high lead to obesity when physical activity decreases and food becomes plentiful.*

Another factor that has contributed to the recent rise in obesity in the United States is the decrease in the number of people who smoke. As people stop smoking, their metabolic rate slows and their food intake tends to increase. In order to avoid weight gain with smoking cessation, an increase in exercise is usually necessary. It is estimated that over the past ten years, 25 percent of the increase in overweight for men and 16 percent of the increase in overweight for women can be explained by smoking cessation.[9]

The Role of Behavior

Do overweight individuals actually eat more or do they use less energy? This has been a difficult question to answer because people do not report their food intake accurately, and the very act of reporting can change the eating pattern. A method called the "doubly labeled water method" allows researchers to accurately measure energy expenditure.[10] In the absence of weight gain or loss, calories consumed should equal calories burned. Researchers found significant differences between the food intake people report versus the energy they expend, with particularly large discrepancies in obese individuals. When energy used in both lean and obese women was measured, the average energy expenditure was higher in the obese group and the basal metabolic rates were identical.[11] This suggests that *obesity is not caused by a reduction in basal metabolism, resulting in fewer calories being burned for energy*. Similar results were found in a study of obese and nonobese adolescents.[12] Basal metabolic rate in both groups depended upon lean body mass, was greater in males than females, and was also greater in the obese group. Obese adolescents expended more energy.

These results suggest that maintaining overweight is a result of increased food consumption.[13] This doesn't necessarily mean that an overweight person is overeating. She may simply be taking in an appropriate amount of calories to produce adequate energy for her body weight.

The Role of the Set Point

In recent years, studies on both rats and humans has supported the concept of a physiological "set point" for body weight.[14] This means that *the body adjusts its food intake and its energy use to maintain a specific weight, and resists both significant weight loss and weight gain.*

How does this process work? In experimental animals, placed on a reduced-calorie diet, two things happen. The basal metabolic rate decreases by an amount much larger than would be expected merely on the basis of the weight loss. Thus, fewer calories are required to maintain each gram of tissue than were needed when the animal was at its usual weight. Second, as soon as the animal is allowed to eat what it wants, it automatically increases its food intake until its previous weight is achieved. The reverse adjustment is seen when animals are force-fed to gain weight. Their energy use increases disproportionately.

For example, studies of a group of obese rats called Zucker rats demonstrated that a weight loss of 6 percent caused the energy needs in these animals to decline to a level equal to that of Zucker rats weighing less than half as much.

This suggests a coordinated adjustment in both food intake and energy use, aimed at maintaining a constant and set body weight, and also implies that overweight may be the natural, normal state for some individuals.

It does appear, at least in animals, that a persistent high-fat diet can elevate the set point. When rats are initially fed a high-fat diet, they compensate by increasing their energy requirements to avoid gaining weight. However, if they stay on a high-fat diet for more than six months, weight gain becomes irreversible, and the animal adjusts its energy use to maintain the higher weight. This increased set point seems to be due to a combination of an increased number of fat cells, with more fat in each cell. When the animal's diet is restricted and it is forced to lose weight, each fat cell becomes smaller, but the total number of fat cells does not change.

How much of this rat research can be applied to humans? It appears that we function in a similar fashion, adjusting our metabolism in response to calorie restriction. One study demonstrated that after undergoing weight loss, an obese group of patients required fewer calories to maintain their weight than a control group weighing 60 percent less. Furthermore, this is not a temporary effect. People who had succeeded in maintaining their weight loss for four to six years still had dramatically reduced energy requirements.[15]

From the point of view of someone attempting to lose weight, this is not good news. It implies that it is often a losing battle. Maintaining weight loss long-term may require a lifetime of restricting eating, feeling hungry, and increasing exercise.

What do we actually know about the factors that determine an individual's set point? Animal studies suggest that a part of the brain called the hypothalamus may be in control of this function. It may also be that appetite suppressing "diet pills" actually function by resetting the set point to a lower weight level. Considerably more research needs to be done to sort out the mechanisms that actually regulate the set point so that we can have an opportunity to adjust it.

The Role of Leptin

In 1995 researchers discovered a gene in mice that appeared to be linked to weight control. This gene produced a strand of messenger RNA, which was named leptin. Leptin, in turn, directed the production of a protein consisting of 167 amino acids. When leptin was given to a strain of very obese mice, lacking the leptin gene, the mice lost 30 percent of their weight. They also exercised more and ate less.

This remarkable finding sparked considerable publicity in the media, as well as enormous research interest in the university and pharmaceutical communities. Had we finally found the magic bullet that would allow for effortless weight loss?

Leptin was rapidly discovered to be present in humans, and it became the subject of an enormous amount of research.[16] It became clear that it was not merely an antiobesity substance, but had a complex role in regulating many other endocrine processes. A full discussion of its many functions is beyond the scope of this book. However, we can review what we currently know about leptin and weight.

Leptin levels increase with increasing fat and overfeeding, and decrease with prolonged fasting. Women appear to have higher leptin levels than men.[17] In order for a protein to affect a tissue in the body, that tissue must have a receptor to which the protein can bind. Receptors for the leptin protein exist in many areas of the brain. Leptin appears to affect many different chemicals produced by the hypothalamus of the brain. These substances are involved in regulating appetite.

Because of the effects of leptin on obese mice, it was initially hoped that we would discover that obese humans were leptin deficient, and that replacing leptin would cause them to lose weight. Unfortunately, this turned out not to be the case. There are rare individuals who have a mutation in the leptin gene and are deficient, but the majority of overweight individuals have high levels of leptin. This suggests that they are resistant to the actions of leptin. The mechanism of this resistance is the subject of much active research.

A number of ongoing clinical trials are looking at whether leptin can help humans to lose weight. Are obese humans completely resistant to leptin or do they simply need an increased dose to respond? What is the best way to administer leptin and what is the correct dose?

In animals such as the rat, dog, and monkey, leptin administration definitely causes weight loss. Researchers are now looking at whether leptin is safe to administer to people. Thus far, no significant adverse side effects have been noted.[18] Definite weight loss was seen when leptin was used in combination with dietary restriction. The amount of weight loss was comparable to that seen with other drugs and appeared to plateau at about six months. *Long-term clinical trials are now under way, and it remains to be seen whether leptin will prove to be a new and valuable tool in the dieter's armamentarium.*

The Role of Ghrelin

The newest hormone on the block, and one which has received great media attention of late, is *Ghrelin*. Ghrelin is made in the stomach and duodenum and has been noted to rise prior to meals and fall after every meal, a pattern suggesting that it may be important in the regulation of appetite.[19] Ghrelin levels were measured in a group of obese individuals before and after a 17 percent weight loss. The hormone level increased 24 percent in the subjects who had lost weight, such that the lowest levels of ghrelin after weight loss were only slightly lower than the highest levels prior to weight loss. This suggests that ghrelin may play a role in increasing appetite to maintain prior body weight after dieting. On the other hand, individuals who had undergone gastric bypass surgery and lost weight were noted to have significantly decreased ghrelin levels, and those levels did not fluctuate before and after meals. Interestingly, people who have undergone gastric bypass succeed in losing large amounts of weight, and in maintaining that weight loss without experiencing significant hunger. It is possible that the lowered levels of ghrelin may be an important factor in weight loss after bypass and that drugs developed to block the effects of ghrelin may soon be developed and tested as another hopeful tool in the dieter's quest.

The Role of Drugs

Antiobesity drugs should not be used during pregnancy. Having said that, it is worthwhile exploring some of the information on the use of these drugs in the nonpregnant state. In 1992 a series of papers were published demonstrating that individuals treated with a combination of fenfluramine and phentermine lost more weight and maintained it for a longer time than a control group undergoing the same diet and exercise program.[20] It was pointed out that physicians have always viewed "diet pills" as a crutch for the weak-willed and have used them only sparingly to help start a diet program. Yet these same physicians would not hesitate to start their patients on long-term therapy for hypertension, diabetes, or thyroid deficiency. *Perhaps we needed to rethink our view of obesity and consider it as a medical condition requiring long-term drug therapy.*

In a remarkably short time Fen/Phen clinics proliferated all over the country and millions of people were using these drugs to diet. Unfortunately, fenfluramine was found to cause heart valve damage and was taken off the market. However, the question of whether drugs can and should be used to reset an individual's set point and continued for long-term weight maintenance remains controversial.

Currently only two drugs on the market are approved for long-term use, sibutramine and orlistat.[21] Sibutramine raises levels of serotonin and norepinephrine, thereby reducing appetite. Orlistat decreases the proportion of fat that is actually digested and results in much of it being excreted in the stool. An unpleasant side effect can be diarrhea accompanying any high-fat splurge. Both these drugs appear to be helpful in maintaining modest weight loss.

Weight-Loss Strategies and Their Results

As is no doubt apparent from the information in this chapter, the most difficult part of losing weight is maintaining the loss. The mainstay of weight-loss therapies has been a combination of low-calorie diets, exercise, and behavior modification. This approach teaches women not only what to eat, but where, when, and under what circumstances. The second half of this book is devoted to some of these strategies, targeted specifically to women who want to be pregnant or who have recently delivered.

Unfortunately, study after study has shown that most overweight individuals regain 35 to 50 percent of their weight loss within one year, and most people regain all of it within five years.[22] This has taught us that weight loss cannot be considered as a short-term project. Long-term, chronic maintenance is as important as initial loss. Furthermore, the goal of reaching an "ideal weight" or appearance may be unrealistic. The National Institute of Health currently recommends that *a realistic goal for treatment of overweight is a 10 percent loss within six months followed by a weight maintenance program. This is because losses of 5 to 10 percent of body weight make significant differences in hypertension, diabetes, and overall health.*[23]

There are no miracle diets or weight-loss programs. We can, however, learn to eat prior, during, and after pregnancy in a way that will optimize health for ourselves and for our babies.

Body Mass Index

Weight (pounds)   Height (Inches)

Weight	60	61	62	63	64	65	66	67	68	69
125	24	24	23	22	22	21	20	20	19	18
130	25	25	24	23	22	22	21	20	20	19
135	26	26	25	24	23	23	22	21	21	20
140	27	27	26	25	24	23	23	22	21	21
145	28	27	27	26	25	24	23	23	22	21
150	29	28	27	27	26	25	24	24	23	22
155	30	29	28	28	27	26	25	24	24	23
160	31	30	29	28	28	27	26	25	24	24
165	32	31	30	39	38	38	37	36	35	24
170	33	32	31	30	29	28	27	27	26	25
175	34	33	32	31	30	29	28	27	27	26
180	35	34	33	32	31	30	29	28	27	27
185	36	35	34	33	32	31	30	29	28	27
190	37	36	35	34	33	32	31	30	29	28
195	38	37	36	35	34	33	32	31	30	29
200	39	38	37	36	34	33	32	31	30	30
205	40	39	38	36	35	34	33	32	31	30
210	41	40	38	37	36	35	34	33	32	31
215	42	41	39	38	37	36	35	34	33	32
220	43	42	40	39	38	37	36	35	34	33
225	44	43	41	40	39	38	36	35	34	33
230	45	44	42	41	40	38	37	36	35	34
235	46	44	43	42	40	39	38	37	36	35
240	47	45	44	43	41	40	39	38	37	36
245	48	46	45	43	42	41	40	38	37	36
250	49	47	46	44	43	42	40	39	38	37
255	50	48	47	45	44	43	41	40	39	38
260	51	49	48	46	45	43	42	41	40	38
265	52	50	49	47	46	44	43	42	40	39
270	53	51	49	48	46	45	44	42	41	40
275	54	52	50	49	47	46	44	43	42	41
280	55	53	51	50	48	47	45	44	43	41
285	56	54	52	51	49	48	46	45	43	42
290	57	55	53	51	50	48	47	46	44	43
295	58	56	54	52	51	49	48	46	45	44
300	59	57	55	53	52	50	49	47	46	44

Great Expectations

Fertility and Weight

t has long been known that weight extremes, in either direction, can disrupt ovulation and lead to problems with conception. An understanding of the complex relationship between your weight and fertility is a first step in tackling potential infertility and achieving a normal pregnancy.

In order to understand how excess weight can cause reproductive problems, it is important to learn about the delicate balancing act that occurs during the menstrual cycle in which five major hormones interact with one another.

GnRF is a hormone produced by a part of your brain called the hypothalamus and carried by your bloodstream directly to the pituitary gland, where it stimulates the pituitary to produce *LH* and *FSH*. LH acts on your ovary to produce *estradiol* (the most important form of estrogen) and progesterone. Your ovary contains thousands of immature eggs, which must grow and ripen in order to be fertilized. FSH is responsible for stimulation of the egg and development of a structure called a follicle, a small cyst, within the ovary, which contains, and ultimately releases, the fully matured egg.

At any given time during the cycle, a process called *feedback* controls the quantities of these five hormones. Positive feedback means that as the level of one hormone rises, it causes the level of another hormone to rise as well. Negative feedback means that rising levels of one hormone will cause a decrease in the production of another.

At the beginning of your cycle, GnRF stimulates your pituitary to produce low levels of LH and FSH. These in turn stimulate your ovaries to produce estradiol, beginning the process of ripening a follicle. During the first week of your cycle, estradiol levels begin to climb and peak just before ovulation. The time from menstruation to ovulation is called the *follicular phase*.

Estradiol and FSH have a negative feedback relationship. As the estradiol levels rise, FSH begins to decrease. The relationship between estradiol and LH is more complex. At low levels of estradiol, negative feedback takes place. However, as the levels of estradiol rise, this changes to positive feedback. As estradiol levels peak, your pituitary releases a large surge of LH, and it is this *LH surge* that signals your ovary to release the ripened egg. Ovulation usually takes place within twenty-four to thirty-six hours after the LH rises.

As soon as you ovulate, your ovary begins to produce progesterone. This second half of your cycle is called the *luteal phase*. High levels of progesterone cause a decrease in LH production. If you do not become pregnant, progesterone levels begin to fall ten or twelve days after ovulation, and within another two to three days of the cycle, all of the hormones are at their lowest point. These low levels of hormones tell your hypothalamus that it is time to begin the whole cycle over again.

During the course of this cycle, both estradiol and progesterone act upon the lining of your uterus, the endometrium.

Estradiol causes the endometrium to grow. Progesterone stimulates the blood vessel supply, preparing the lining to nourish a pregnancy. If fertilization occurs, progesterone continues to be produced by your ovary, and the lining remains stable and continues to thicken. If there is no pregnancy, the drop in estradiol and progesterone at the end of the cycle causes your lining to break down and bleed or menstruate.

Obviously there are many places in this complex pathway where things can go wrong and interfere with normal ovulation, but what does weight have to do with it?

Weight and the Onset of Menstruation

Weight enters the picture at the very beginning, at the onset of puberty. During childhood your levels of LH and FSH are low and constant. As puberty approaches, surges of LH begin to be released during sleep, followed by a pattern of cyclic pulses during the day. This pattern eventually evolves to the familiar adult pattern, which stimulates the production of estradiol and progesterone.[1] This is followed by your first menstrual period.

It is interesting to note that the age at which girls first menstruate has been gradually decreasing over the past 160 years in the Western world. In Norway, in 1840, the average age was seventeen. By 1960 the age was thirteen. In the United States, in 1900, girls menstruated at an average age of fourteen. By 1960 the age had decreased to 12.6.[2] It is widely believed that this decrease in the age of first menses is due to better nutrition, so that girls reach a minimum body weight and body-fat content earlier. The body weight and fat content are required to trigger the hormonal changes.

LH begins to increase at a weight of 77 pounds and when the amount of body fat reaches 20 pounds. Its major increase occurs at 100 pounds, at which time there is also a marked increase in the production of estradiol. FSH behaves similarly.[3] Thus, heavier teenagers will menstruate much earlier than thin, physically active girls with low body fat. The ratio of body weight to body fat changes as a girl matures. At the time of puberty, the ratio is 5:1. By the time of the first period, it becomes 3:1. As girls mature they accumulate fat at a faster rate than lean body mass. At the onset of menstruation, fat constitutes approximately 22 percent of the total body weight. By the age of eighteen, for most women, the percentage of body fat is 26 to 28 percent.[4]

Once established, your normal menstrual cycle is to some extent body-fat dependent, and can be disrupted by extremes of both weight loss and weight gain. When you diet, much of your weight loss is fat. Thus, a relatively small percentage loss of body weight can represent a large percentage of total body fat, particularly if you are in the normal-weight range to begin with. For example, if a normal weight woman loses 10 to 15 percent of her weight, she is losing 33 percent of her body fat. This can shift her percentage of body fat back to the prepubertal stage, and lead to subsequent menstrual abnormalities.[5]

The Effects of Obesity on Ovulation and Estrogen Production

Endocrine abnormalities that affect ovulation and menstruation can occur in women who are obese. It is important to distinguish those women who are truly obese from those who are merely overweight. This is done using the BMI or body mass index, defined in the previous chapter.

For women in the twenty-to-twenty-nine-year age group, 85 percent have a BMI less than 27.3.[6] Most studies that examine medical problems associated with obesity use a BMI greater than 27 to define their obese population. This number is not arbitrary but reflects the point at which excess fat has been demonstrated to become a health risk. Some individuals with a high BMI have excess weight due to muscle mass rather than fat, but for those of us who are not bodybuilders, the BMI is a useful tool.

If you are obese, or significantly overweight, and experiencing problems with fertility, the reason is most likely to be failure to ovulate. Estrogen levels in overweight women are elevated or normal. So why should an overweight woman experience ovulation problems?

Estradiol is not the only estrogen synthesized in humans. *Estrone*, a weak estrogen, is produced from a hormone called androstenedione, made by your adrenal gland. In order for the chemical reaction converting androstenedione to estrone to take place, a specialized protein called an enzyme is required. The enzyme needed for this particular reaction exists in fat cells. Thus, the more fat cells you have, the more estrone you make. Estrone can then be converted to estradiol. Remember that estradiol in the bloodstream exerts a negative feedback on FSH. This interferes with the growth of the follicle so that your egg does not ripen on schedule and ovulation does not take place.

Obesity and Polycystic Ovary Syndrome

Some obese women have an endocrine disorder called polycystic ovary syndrome, abbreviated as *PCO*. If you have this disorder, you have irregular menses without ovulation and enlarged ovaries with large numbers of unruptured follicle cysts. Approximately 35 to 50 percent of women with PCO are obese and many have excess facial and body hair. The endocrine abnormalities and their relationships are very complex and not necessarily present consistently in all women with the disease. However, we can summarize the most common end results.

Women with PCO have elevated levels of LH and decreased levels of FSH. The elevated LH levels lead to increased production of estradiol and testosterone. The high estrogen levels, through their negative-feedback effect, result in decreased FSH and inadequate stimulation of the follicle and egg. Women with PCO have enlarged ovaries with many unruptured small follicle cysts because the follicles never become mature enough to release the egg; hence the name polycystic ovary syndrome. The increased levels of testosterone account for unsightly facial and body hair and may also produce acne. The high levels of estrogen stimulate the uterine lining to thicken. Because ovulation does not take place, and progesterone is not produced, there is no regular monthly shedding of the lining. Eventually, when the lining becomes so thick that it is unstable, some of it will break off, causing bleeding. You may have extremely heavy prolonged periods or daily spotting that lasts for many days or weeks. In addition, continuously stimulating the same endometrial lining cells with estrogen can lead to precancerous abnormalities.

Over the past ten years, an additional factor has been discovered in this complex endocrine abnormality. Women with PCO have been found to have increased *insulin resistance*.[7] What does that mean and what are the implications for therapy? Insulin, a hormone produced by the pancreas, takes glucose from the bloodstream and transfers it inside our cells, where it can be metabolized for energy. If you are resistant to insulin, a larger quantity is necessary to do the work, and women with insulin resistance have higher insulin levels. The insulin also acts on your ovaries, making them more sensitive to LH and resulting in increased production of testosterone. Finally, the insulin acts on your liver, decreasing the production of a protein whose function is to bind estradiol and testosterone. In the bound form, these hormones are inactive. Thus the ultimate effect of the increased insulin is to increase the active, unbound form of estradiol and testosterone, interfering with ovulation.

Obese women with PCO are at significant risk of developing *adult onset diabetes* in their forties and fifties.[8] In one study, 80 percent of obese women who were also adult diabetics were found to have polycystic ovaries on ultrasound. These findings suggest that all obese women with PCO should have regular glucose tests and that all young adult diabetics should be evaluated for PCO.

Treatment of Women with PCO

If you have been diagnosed with PCO, the goal of treatment is to restore normal periods, break the cycle of elevated hormones, and induce ovulation when you wish to become pregnant. A combination of birth-control pills and antiandrogen drugs has been the mainstay of therapy. Birth control pills cause regular shedding of uterine lining, controlling the abnormal bleeding. They also stimulate the liver to produce more of the protein that binds testosterone, decreasing acne and growth of facial hair. However, they are not useful when you want to become pregnant.

Recently, several authors have suggested that drugs called *insulin sensitizing agents* may improve symptoms and increase pregnancy rates in women with PCO by lowering insulin levels.[9] A drug called Metformin has been the subject of several studies. One study used Metformin against a placebo and found that women on the drug had an increased frequency of menstruation and decreased insulin levels and blood sugar levels.[10] Another evaluated Metformin against a birth-control pill. The women on Metformin had improved menses, lost weight, and had decreased blood sugar and insulin. The women on birth-control pills showed more improvement in androgen-related symptoms such as acne.[11] Yet another study looked at Metformin in combination with a very low-calorie diet against a placebo. In that study both cycles and excess hair were improved on the drug.[12]

Weight loss alone, without drugs, can cause improvement in the endocrine imbalance. Women with PCO on a very low calorie weight loss diet were noted to have decreased LH concentration,[13] and women who lost more than 5 percent of their body weight had a 70 percent spontaneous conception rate.[14]

What Can Be Done to Achieve Pregnancy in Obese Women?

If you are obese, the most common cause of infertility is simply failure to ovulate. Your doctor can attempt to correct some of the endocrine abnormalities and restore normal spontaneous menstrual cycles or can induce ovulation.

A group of sixty-seven obese women who were not ovulating agreed to participate in a supervised weight loss and exercise program. Over a six-month period these women lost an average of 22 pounds. Of these women, sixty resumed normal ovulation and fifty-two became pregnant with no intervention other than weight loss.[15]

Induction of ovulation will usually restore fertility if your only problem is ovulation related. There are two strategies for stimulating ovulation. The easiest is to take a drug called clomiphene (Clomid). Clomid fools your hypothalamus into thinking that the level of estradiol in your circulation is low. Your hypothalamus then stimulates your pituitary to produce more FSH and LH. This works well for normal-weight or obese women. The drug is easy to use, not too expensive, and has a lower rate of multiple pregnancy than the alternative.

If you do not respond to Clomid, the most effective way to induce ovulation is with Pergonal (a mixture of FSH and LH) or with pure FSH. These drugs are given daily as a shot, and your estrogen level is monitored. Ultrasounds are performed to determine the number and size of the follicles produced. When the estrogen level and follicle size are adequate, ovulation is induced. You then have intercourse at home, or artificial insemination can be performed the same day in the physician's office.

In a study of 333 women undergoing ovulation induction with Pergonal followed by in vitro fertilization, 76 were obese (BMI of 27.9 or above). Compared to controls, there was no difference in the pregnancy rate, implantation rate and miscarriage rate.[16] A similar study of women undergoing in vitro fertilization with a body mass greater than 30 kg/m^2 found that a larger quantity of Pergonal was required to produce multiple ovulations.[17]

You will usually not need to proceed to in vitro fertilization if your only problem is simply lack of ovulation. In vitro techniques are usually performed for women who have blocked fallopian tubes or a husband with a very low sperm count.

Since weight loss alone can successfully restore ovulation in many women, you might want to try it first. However, if you have repeatedly tried and failed to lose weight, it is reassuring to know that ovulation induction is likely to be successful and to result in a pregnancy.

Obesity and Miscarriages

A number of studies have suggested that women who are overweight or obese have an increased rate of spontaneous pregnancy loss. A study of 9,239 women looked at miscarriage rate against BMI.[18] Normal-weight women (BMI = 19 – 24.9) had a miscarriage rate of 11 percent. Overweight women (BMI =

25 – 27.9) had a 14 percent rate, while women with a BMI greater than 28 lost 15 percent of their early pregnancies. In another study, women who were overweight and had PCO had a 47 percent pregnancy loss compared with thin women with PCO who had a 27 percent loss rate.[19] A third study examined the outcome of in vitro fertilization procedures in obese versus thin women. They found that fewer eggs were collected per cycle and that there was an increased loss rate at six weeks gestation; 22 percent for obese women (BMI greater than 25) vs. 12 percent for thin women.[20] Although the actual numbers are variable, the trend seems clear. Increased weight appears correlated with a higher miscarriage risk.

Must an Obese Woman Lose Weight Before Attempting Pregnancy?

The answer to this question depends on how obese one is and whether there are preexisting medical conditions such as diabetes and hypertension, which will make the pregnancy much more difficult and which could improve substantially with weight loss. If you are significantly overweight, you may already have put many aspects of your life on hold while attempting weight loss. It is common to hear an overweight woman say that she won't buy new clothes, attempt to date, go on vacation anyplace that requires wearing a bathing suit, or get pregnant until she loses weight. "Losing weight" in her mind may be synonymous with "being thin" and may involve the loss of 50, 75, or 100 pounds, a daunting, overwhelming, and time-consuming project that she has no doubt attempted many times in her life. The good news is that weight loss of this magnitude is not necessary for a healthy successful pregnancy! A weight loss of 5 to 10 percent could be all that it takes to restore normal ovulation, lower blood pressure, and improve adult onset diabetes. Your desirable weight gain in pregnancy, depending upon your start-ing weight, is 15 to 30 pounds. Losing this amount ahead of time will reduce the cardiovascular strain imposed by preg-nancy. Again, you need to evaluate your BMI and medical con-dition with your physician to set an individual and achievable prepregnancy weight-loss goal. If you consider yourself over-weight but do not meet the medical criteria for obesity, weight loss may not be necessary at all.

Issues Associated with Unplanned Pregnancy

Unfortunately, not all pregnancies are carefully planned in advance. If your periods are very irregular or nonexistent, you may be careless about birth control, assuming you can't become pregnant without active intervention. Because a simple missed period is not a red flag, you may ignore the signs and symptoms of pregnancy until the pregnancy is advanced. Even then, you may visit your doctor for relief of symptoms you assume have some other cause. Once you discover you are pregnant, you need to decide the best course for you.

For some women, there is no choice about whether or not to remain pregnant. Their religious beliefs or personal morals pro-hibit them from even considering abortion. Others are forced to examine their most deeply held feelings about parenthood. Their struggle is complicated by the question of what effect their obesity might have on the health of a child.

Having the facts is crucial to making the right decision. Some of these facts are contained in this book. However, general information should be interpreted by a skilled physician and applied individually to each woman. Consultation with a gyne-cologist, internist, and nutritionist can help you attain a medical perspective on your issues and define the steps that you need to take if your pregnancy is to continue and be successful.

If you decide to proceed with an unplanned pregnancy, then immediate nutritional intervention is important. Much of the detailed nutritional information for eating well, when pregnant, can be found in Section II of this book. It should be combined with a consultation with a certified dietitian in order to construct an individualized diet plan.

A Strategy for Success

Throughout this book the authors emphasize the importance of a team approach to successful pregnancy. Think of pregnancy as an athletic event that imposes new fitness demands on the body. The coaches are the obstetrician and nutritionist. Each of them brings a different prospective and a unique set of skills to the same problem. Make certain that they are both available and on the team. You have made a commitment to a successful pregnancy and you need to be surrounded by people who are supportive of your efforts. The coaches need to communicate with one another about the pregnancy and pool their expertise. Solicit support and positive reinforcement from family, friends, and of course, the father-to-be.

In the next chapter we will discuss the effects of obesity on pregnancy and will examine some of the complications that can occur if unhealthy eating behaviors are not changed. We will explain how and why these complications arise and how they are handled.

Chapter Three

Fetus vs. Fat

The Point of Diminishing Returns

One of the first questions every pregnant woman asks her doctor is "how much weight should I gain?" Women want to eat in a healthy manner to provide adequate nutrition for their growing babies, but no one wants to end her pregnancy with an extra 20 pounds adorning her hips. It turns out that the answer to the above question depends to a large extent on a woman's prepregnancy weight.

We tell our patients who are underweight and normal weight that dieting during pregnancy is a bad idea. The calories go first to the mother, and the baby gets the leftovers. Therefore, a thin woman who restricts her calories will wind up with a baby that is small or even growth retarded. If you are overweight or obese (BMI > 30), however, the situation is different. You have plenty of extra energy stored in your fat cells and do not need to increase your calories nearly as much. You can produce a normal weight, healthy baby with a significantly smaller weight gain.

The Institute of Medicine has issued guidelines over the years for appropriate pregnancy weight gain. The 1990 guidelines suggest the following weight gains based on BMI.[1]

BMI	Recommended Weight Gain
< 19.8	28–40 lbs.
19.8–26	25–35 lbs.
26.1–29	15–25 lbs.
> 29	at least 15 lbs.

Thus, if you are overweight or obese, you should gain a minimum of 15 pounds and not more than 25 pounds during the course of your pregnancy.

What kind of evidence do we have that these recommendations are appropriate? Numerous studies have attempted to estimate the point of diminishing returns, to correlate obstetrical complications with weight gain, and to determine which women are at risk for retaining weight after pregnancy. Not all of the weight gain of pregnancy goes directly to the baby. You need to make a placenta, grow a very large uterus, expand your breast tissue, and manufacture about six pints of new blood to support the growing baby and extra tissues. Most of this weight is lost rapidly, shortly after delivery.

A study done at the University of Michigan analyzed maternal weight gain and tried to estimate the proportion of weight that is needed for the pregnancy vs. excess retained weight. Researchers measured each woman's prepregnancy weight, the weight of her baby, and her postpartum weight two days after delivery. They defined "retained weight" as postpartum weight minus prepregnancy weight. They found, in their sample, that for every pound of retained weight, normal-weight women increased their baby's weight by .25 oz and obese women increased their baby's weight by only .08 oz. Furthermore, in women who gained more than the recommended guidelines, both birth weight and retained weight were increased. In the sample of normal-weight women, birth weight increased 5.9 percent at the price of 13 pounds of retained weight. For obese women, birth weight increased a mere .3 percent, while retained weight averaged 18 pounds. Clearly, in obese women, the point of diminishing returns occurs sooner than it does in normal-weight women.[2]

How much of the total weight gain is water and how much is body fat in women who adhere to the Institute of Medicine guidelines? A group from Columbia University measured body composition in 200 women at fourteen and thirty-seven weeks gestation. Body water gain did not differ between underweight, normal weight, overweight, and obese women. Overweight and obese women had little or no change in body fat, provided they stayed within the Institute of Medicine guidelines.[3]

What kinds of complications can be expected in overweight women when they become pregnant, and to what extent are those complications related to the amount of weight gained during the pregnancy? There have been a very large number of studies that have demonstrated, unequivocally, that *overweight and obese women are at significantly higher risk for a large number of serious complications during pregnancy, during labor and delivery, and postpartum.* Much of this evidence, as well as the specific complications, will be discussed in later chapters.

The question we wish to address now is, which complications are directly related to the amount of pregnancy weight gain? According to a study of complications and pregnancy weight gain in 683 obese and 660 normal-weight women, although obese women had a much higher rate of overall complications, the complications did not correlate with how much weight they gained during their pregnancies. Women who lost weight or did not gain any weight were more likely to deliver infants under 6.6 pounds—small for their gestational age. Women who gained more than 35 pounds were twice as likely to deliver very large babies, 8.8 pounds or above, and to put themselves at increased risk for a cesarean section.[4] A similar study also found that the complication rate was not affected by the actual pregnancy weight gain, but that women who gained more than 25 pounds had excessively large babies. The conclusion was that morbidly obese women should not gain more than 25 pounds during pregnancy.[5]

The most important point to be retained from these studies is that you are at risk for increased complications if you are overweight or obese at the time you become pregnant, and this is true regardless of the amount of weight you gain during pregnancy.

Finally, we should explore the question of whether pregnancy predisposes a woman to becoming overweight in later life, and which women are at particular risk for this. Two studies are particularly pertinent to this question, one from Sweden and a second from Kaiser, a large HMO. The Kaiser study, which followed 1,300 women through two pregnancies, found that the women at highest risk of becoming overweight after pregnancy were young (twenty-four to thirty), had gained an excessive amount of weight during their pregnancies, had menstruated at a young age (< 12), and had a short interval from their first period to their first birth. Caucasian women were 4.5 times as likely to become overweight as Asian women.[6] The Swedish study found that the factor that most strongly predicted retention of pregnancy weight was the weight increase during pregnancy. In addition, women who had stopped smoking during their pregnancy, and who reported significant lifestyle changes with respect to physical activity and eating habits, were more likely to retain weight.[7] Clearly, pregnancy can be a triggering event that leads to future overweight and obesity.

In the following chapters we will examine the complications that can occur in obese women both during and after pregnancy, and discuss how these complications can be managed so that both mother and child are healthy.

Chapter Four

The Nine-Month Weight

Pregnancy Complications

in Obese Women

Unfortunately, even with excellent prenatal care, mothers who are overweight or obese are subject to an increased risk of a myriad of pregnancy complications. *These include chronic hypertension, pregnancy-induced hypertension, preeclampsia, diabetes, gestational diabetes, stillbirth, and an increase in congenital abnormalities.* In the following chapter we will examine the medical evidence for this statement and discuss the most common complications in detail. This chapter is not meant to frighten you. The majority of plus-sized women will have normal, uneventful pregnancies. However, because overweight women are at increased risk, it is important to be alert and prepared. Complications that are diagnosed early by your physician and managed carefully should not prevent you from having a healthy baby.

The Weight of the Evidence

Numerous studies have been performed attempting to correlate maternal prepregnancy BMI with various complications during pregnancy. Among the more recent, a very large study examined 96,801 live birth certificates from the state of Washington during the years 1992 to 1996 and found that with increasing BMI there was a consistent increase in gestational diabetes, preeclampsia, and eclampsia. This was true for both overweight (BMI > 25, < 30) and obese (BMI > 30) women. These women were also at higher risk for premature delivery (< 37 weeks), cesarean section, and for a twofold increase in infant death within one year of birth. When women with gestational diabetes, prepregnancy diabetes and hypertension, preeclampsia, and eclampsia were eliminated from the calculation, the data still showed that overweight and obesity alone increased the risk for premature delivery, cesarean section, and infant death. *This study was particularly important because it demonstrated that not only markedly obese women, but also overweight women (BMI > 25) were at risk for all these complications.*[1]

A study of obese Israeli women, matched with a control group, also demonstrated increased gestational diabetes, pregnancy-induced hypertension, labor induction, cesarean section, and very large infants.[2] Another group of researchers demonstrated similar results in 613 morbidly obese women (BMI > 35) and 11,313 normal-weight controls.[3] These represent only a few of the many pieces of evidence in the medical literature demonstrating that increased weight causes increased risk.

Obesity and Congenital Abnormalities

A number of congenital abnormalities, not due to chromosome or genetic defects, have been shown to occur at increased levels in infants of obese mothers.

The state of California has a comprehensive screening program that looks for an abnormality called a *neural tube defect (NTD)*. The neural tube is a primitive structure found in the embryo that develops into the brain and spinal cord. When things go wrong, a number of defects can develop, the most common of which are *spina bifida* and *anencephaly*. In spina bifida, there is incomplete closure of the spinal cord, resulting in various neurological defects, depending on the location of the abnormality. All of the nerves that come out of the spinal cord below the level of the defect are involved. A defect that is below the waist can result in leg paralysis and lack of control of bowel and bladder. A defect that is high, in the region of the chest or just below the neck, can result in complete paralysis of all the limbs and breathing problems. In anencephaly, the brain itself fails to develop. This results in stillbirth or death within a few days after birth.

Higher levels of a protein called *alpha fetoprotein* are present in the maternal blood of women who are carrying a baby with a neural tube defect. In California, all pregnant women receive a blood test measuring this protein as well as the hormones HCG and estriol. The test is called the Triple Screen. If you have an elevated alpha fetoprotein level, this does not necessarily mean that your baby has an NTD. Other factors can be involved. However, the blood test serves to identify a group of women who are at higher risk and who must be examined more closely.

If you have an elevated alpha fetoprotein, the next step is to have an amniocentesis, which looks for any genetic abnormalities, and a careful ultrasound by a trained perinatal ultrasonographer, examining the brain and spine for evidence of a neural tube problem. Although no imaging technique is 100 percent accurate, ultrasound does an excellent job of identifying these defects. If an NTD is identified, you and your husband will normally undergo counseling to inform you of the handicaps that can be expected from the location of the spina bifida or brain defect that is diagnosed. Based on this information, and your own convictions about abortion, you can then decide whether to continue or terminate the pregnancy.

The largest study on this subject examined the risk for NTD among obese women (BMI > 29).[4] Interviews were done with 538 women who had been diagnosed with an NTD, including both those who terminated and those who chose not to. This group was matched with a control group of mothers who had normal infants. *Obese women had 1.9 times the risk of a pregnancy with a neural tube defect*. This risk was greater for spina bifida than for anencephaly.

Why should obesity be associated with this increased risk? We know that prenatal use of folic acid (.4 mg daily) lowers the risk for an NTD in the general population. We routinely counsel our patients to take folic acid while they are attempting conception. Since this study showed no difference in folic acid intake between obese women and controls, it may be that in overweight women, folic acid loses its protective effect. Perhaps obese women need a larger dose to achieve the same protection. The answer to this question awaits further study.

What about other kinds of congenital, nonchromosomal defects? Data from 22,951 pregnant women was analyzed in order to examine the effects of maternal obesity and diabetes.[5] *In women who are obese, but not diabetic, the overall risk of an abnormality is not increased*. This is also true for women who have preexisting diabetes or gestational diabetes, but are normal weight. *However, certain specific abnormalities are more com-*

monly found in obese women. These include cleft lip or palate, clubfoot, abnormalities in the septum of the heart (the membrane that divides the left and right sides), hydrocephalus (the buildup of fluid in the brain), and abdominal wall hernias. *Women who are both obese and diabetic have 3.1 times the overall risk of having a child who suffers from some sort of congenital defect.*

Most of the congenital abnormalities for which the babies of obese and diabetic women are at risk can be identified by ultrasound. We routinely send our patients to a perinatal ultrasonographer for a structural scan at eighteen to twenty weeks gestation. Fortunately many congenital anomalies associated with obese diabetic women are amenable to surgical correction immediately after birth or during childhood.

The increased risk for nongenetic congenital abnormalities in women who are obese suggests that all significantly overweight mothers should have careful screening with alpha fetoprotein and second trimester ultrasound.

Obesity and the Hypertensive Disorders of Pregnancy

Women who begin their pregnancies overweight or obese are more likely to have preexisting hypertension, to develop pregnancy-induced hypertension (PIH), or to wind up with preeclampsia or eclampsia. These disorders, if not recognized and properly managed, can lead to significant problems, even to life threatening ones, for both mother and baby. Chronic hypertension, PIH, and preeclampsia have been reported in 27 to 35 percent of severely obese women as compared with 3 to 19 percent of normal-weight women.[6, 7]

The Normal Heart Adaptations of Pregnancy

Pregnancy itself causes a variety of normal cardiovascular changes as the heart and blood vessels adapt to the extra load of the developing baby. In a normal pregnancy, blood pressure decreases during the first and second trimesters, usually reaching a minimum at about twenty weeks and then returning to normal levels in the third trimester. The blood volume and metabolic rate increase, causing the heart to work harder, pumping more blood with each contraction and contracting at a higher rate. Blood vessels throughout the body normally relax to lower the resistance against which the heart has to work. The average woman manufactures an extra six pints of blood to meet the needs of the baby and placenta. The chamber of the left ventricle of the heart enlarges to accommodate the larger volume of blood that is being pumped, but in normal pregnancies, the heart wall muscle itself does not thicken in response to the extra load.

Heart Function in Obese Women

In nonpregnant, obese women the heart works harder than in normal-weight women simply to meet the demands of the excess fat for blood and oxygen. Even obese women who do not suffer from high blood pressure have dilated left ventricles with thickened walls.[8] Pregnancy imposes additional strain on the hearts of morbidly obese women. The left atrium increases in size, and the wall of the left ventricle becomes thicker, as does the septum dividing the left and right ventricles.[9]

Defining the Hypertensive Disorders

To begin with, let us describe the measurement of blood pressure and explain what the numbers mean. You will see blood pressure written as two numbers, for example 120/80. The higher number, in this case 120, is called the systolic pressure. It represents the pressure encountered by the heart at the moment it contracts, sending blood into the arteries. The lower number, the diastolic blood pressure, is the pressure of the blood in the vessels when the heart is not contracting. It is influenced by how elastic the blood vessels are. Arteries that dilate easily will result in a low diastolic blood pressure. As arteries age and become clogged with plaques of cholesterol and fat, they harden, and the diastolic blood pressure increases. Physicians like to see blood pressures that are below 140/90.

A woman whose blood pressure is consistently above 140/90 prior to her pregnancy may be said to have *chronic hypertension*. She may or may not be on antihypertensive medications, depending upon how high her blood pressures have been in the past.

A woman who enters pregnancy with normal blood pressure, and who begins to have elevations above 140/90, in the absence of any of the symptoms of preeclampsia, may be said to have *pregnancy-induced hypertension*, abbreviated *PIH*.

Preeclampsia is a common pregnancy disorder, found in 5 to 10 percent of all pregnancies. It can be mild, moderate, or severe. The hallmarks of preeclampsia are hypertension (above 140/90 after twenty weeks gestation), protein in the urine, and edema or generalized swelling.

The most dangerous complication of preeclampsia is the development of *eclampsia*. Women with eclampsia have generalized seizures, either during labor or the twenty-four hours after delivery. Eclampsia can lead to significant complications for both mother and baby, and physicians go to great lengths to manage preeclampsia before it can progress to eclampsia.

The Evidence for Increased Risk in Obese Women

One researcher followed the blood pressures of 249 obese pregnant women and 1,843 controls throughout pregnancy.[10] The obese women had higher pressures throughout pregnancy as well as significantly more PIH. Other studies found that preexisting hypertension was present in 33 percent of women weighing over 300 pounds versus only 5 percent in normal weight women.[11, 12]

Numerous studies have also found that obese women have an increased incidence of preeclampsia[13, 14] and eclampsia.[15, 16, 17] Obese women are 3.5 times more likely to develop severe preeclampsia than normal-weight women.[18]

Diagnosis of the Hypertensive Disorders

The diagnosis of chronic hypertension in pregnancy is normally straightforward. A woman will come to her obstetrician with a history of previously diagnosed high blood pressure, or will be noted to have pressures equal to or above 140/90 during the first trimester. A woman with normal pressure in the first half of pregnancy who then develops blood pressure elevation is said to have pregnancy-induced hypertension. Every single obstetrical examination normally includes measurement of blood pressure. *It is important to be aware of the fact that overweight women with heavy arms must have their pressure measured with a large cuff.* One study looked at three commercially available blood pressure cuffs designed to measure blood pressure at home in obese pregnant women. None of these devices turned out to be accurate.[19]

Preeclampsia is suspected in a woman whose blood pressure is persistently 140/90 and above and who spills at least .3 grams/day of protein in a urine specimen collected over twenty-four hours. Once again, the measurement of urine protein is a routine part of every obstetrical examination. Usually this is done with a dipstick. Protein is characterized as not present, trace, 1+, 2+, or 3+. A protein level of 1+ is suspicious for developing preeclampsia and warrants further testing. As protein leaves the vascular tree through the capillaries and is excreted in the urine, the remaining blood serum becomes less concentrated and leaks out of blood vessels into the surrounding tissue. This causes the edema or swelling so common in preeclamptic women. Feet and ankles swell, fingers become too swollen for rings, and faces look puffy. Edema alone, however, is often found in normal pregnant women, especially in the feet and ankles. This is because the uterus is putting pressure on the vena cava, the major blood vessel that returns blood to the heart from the lower extremities. As blood return slows, excess fluid accumulates in the feet.

Severe preeclampsia is identified by blood pressures of 160/110 or above and 3+ protein in the urine. Symptoms may include persistent headaches, visual disturbances, or pain in the upper abdomen. Laboratory abnormalities may include lowered platelets, prolonged clotting times, elevated liver enzymes, and elevated levels of uric acid. Women with severe preeclampsia are at high risk for seizures and must be managed aggressively and delivered as soon as possible.

Caring for Overweight, Hypertensive Pregnant Women

In pregnant women who are chronically hypertensive, the probability of a bad outcome seems to depend on whether or not preeclampsia develops. Among all pregnancies, the incidence of PIH or superimposed preeclampsia is in the range of 15 to 25 percent. In obese, chronically hypertensive women, as we have seen, the odds of developing preeclampsia are increased.

Physicians have debated whether or not to treat pregnant women with chronic hypertension with medication.[20] One can expect, at least during the first half of pregnancy, that the normal changes will lower blood pressure. A number of studies have divided hypertensive pregnant women into two groups. One group received treatment (drugs to keep blood pressure under 140/90) and the other group had no treatment unless diastolic blood pressure was 110 or above. These studies demonstrated that there was no difference between the groups in the important complications of pregnancy. Treatment with blood-pressure-lowering drugs did not appear to protect women from developing preeclampsia. The worst complications were observed in women who began their pregnancy with severe hypertension. At least half of them developed preeclampsia, and all the truly bad outcomes were found in this group. These included premature deliveries, growth retardation, and fetal death.

When it is necessary to prescribe medication to lower excessively high blood pressure during pregnancy, physicians prefer to use a small number of blood pressure drugs that appear to have no adverse consequences for the baby. These include alpha-methyldopa, labetalol, nifedipine, and apresoline. If you are already taking a medication at the start of your pregnancy, your obstetrician must evaluate the drug for its safety during pregnancy. It may be necessary to stop or to switch medications. Certain classes of blood pressure drugs called beta-blockers and ACE inhibitors are considered unsafe for pregnant women.

Once preeclampsia has been diagnosed, either on its own or together with existing hypertension, the only cure is delivery. The disease, its symptoms, and laboratory abnormalities disappear rapidly after birth. If you are close to term, the solution is simple. Labor may be induced, or if indicated for other reasons, a cesarean section may be performed. It is when preeclampsia develops remote from term, and the baby's lungs are not yet mature, that the dilemma occurs. One would like to prolong the pregnancy, as long as it is safe for the mother, until the baby is mature enough so that neonatal intensive care is unnecessary.

In times past, if you were initially diagnosed with mild preeclampsia, you were admitted to a hospital for laboratory evaluation and complete bed rest.[21] This appeared to be effective in lowering blood pressure and improving infant survival. Adding blood-pressure-lowering medications did not appear to change the outcomes. With the advent of managed care, however, prolonged hospitalization has become less feasible. Subsequent studies questioned the role of bed rest and demonstrated that there was no difference in stillbirth between those women who were hospitalized and those who were treated as outpatients. The key appeared to be careful surveillance of both mother and baby. Now we perform twice-weekly fetal ultrasounds and fetal heart rate testing to assess the baby. If the baby's status deteriorates, you are admitted to the hospital and stabilized. You will have daily blood pressures, urine protein, and fetal movement counts.

If you develop severe preeclampsia, you should be considered for immediate delivery. Your greatest dangers are the development of grand mal seizures or stroke from highly elevated blood pressures. The drug magnesium sulfate has been used successfully for years to prevent seizures in both mild and severe preeclamptics. It is normally administered in a continuous intravenous drip. Extremely high blood pressure can be lowered to acceptable values with appropriate drugs. Once stabilization has occurred, immediate delivery should follow if the pregnancy is close to term. In the premature baby, amniocentesis can be considered to assess fetal lung maturity. Fortunately, the stress of high blood pressure often results in early lung maturation. If the fetus's lungs are not mature, you, your obstetrician, and your perinatologist must carefully weigh the risk to both mother and baby of prolonging the pregnancy. In some cases, testing will show significant deterioration even in the immature fetus, and it will be clear that the baby will be better off delivered. These decisions are clinically complex and very individual. Clear communication of the risks and benefits of each course of action is essential.

Overweight and Diabetic Complications of Pregnancy

Diabetes is a disorder in the metabolism of glucose, the sugar that is the body's primary source of energy. The body takes in complex sugars and carbohydrates, which are then digested and processed to produce glucose. Specialized cells in the pancreas called beta cells produce the protein insulin, the function of which is to carry glucose into the cells, where it is then broken down and converted to energy. Excess glucose is stored in the liver as a substance called glycogen, which can be mobilized and used as needed. If the process is working properly, the concentration of free glucose in the bloodstream is held within a normal range.

There are two distinct types of diabetes. In type 1, or juvenile diabetes, there is damage to the beta cells of the pancreas. The initial insult is believed to be viral, and the body's immune system then makes antibodies that destroy beta cells. As a result, insulin production is impaired and women require daily insulin injections in order to transfer glucose into their cells and to avoid very high blood sugar levels. This type of diabetes is not associated with increased body weight.

Type 2 diabetes, on the other hand, is found much more commonly in overweight adults. The beta cells are able to produce insulin, but the body's tissues are resistant to its action. Thus, a larger amount of insulin is necessary to maintain normal blood sugar levels. Adults with type 2 diabetes have abnormally high insulin levels, and eventually, when the beta cells become exhausted and cannot make additional insulin, elevated blood glucose levels begin to appear. Type 2 diabetes is responsive to diet or to oral medications and does not always require insulin therapy.

Pregnant overweight women are at increased risk for both preexisting type 2 diabetes and for gestational (pregnancy-induced) diabetes.

Understanding Gestational Diabetes

Gestational diabetes is defined as glucose intolerance that is first detected during the course of pregnancy. It is a type 2 diabetes, based on insulin resistance rather than lack of insulin production. A variety of maternal fetal and placental hormones, produced in larger quantities during the latter half of pregnancy, function to raise glucose levels and require greater insulin production. Women who are overweight and insulin resistant to begin with are unable to maintain the necessary insulin levels and end up with elevated glucose.

Diagnosing Gestational Diabetes

All pregnant women should be screened in the second trimester with a *50-gram glucose screen*. This test is usually performed at twenty-eight weeks gestation. You drink the glucose and have your blood drawn an hour later. If the plasma glucose value is equal to or greater than 140 mg/ml, you then require a three-hour glucose tolerance test. This involves drinking a 100-gram glucose drink, and having blood drawn fasting, and one, two, and three hours after ingestion. The American College of Obstetricians and Gynecologists has defined criteria for diagnosing gestational diabetes based on this test. If two or more values are met or exceeded, the diagnosis is made.[22]

Three-Hour Glucose Tolerance Test

Time	Plasma glucose mg/ml
Fasting	95
1 hour	180
2 hour	155
3 hour	140

Because overweight women are at increased risk for gestational diabetes and for preexisting type 2 diabetes, it is a good idea to screen early in pregnancy. If your tests are abnormal in the first trimester, you most likely have previously undiagnosed type 2 diabetes. If your tests are normal in the first trimester, you must still be screened at twenty-eight weeks.

Risks Associated with Gestational Diabetes

Of women whose pregnancies are complicated by diabetes (2 to 3 percent of all pregnancies) about 90 percent have gestational diabetes rather than preexisting type 1 diabetes. This is fortunate because type 1 diabetes leads to a significantly increased risk of miscarriage, congenital abnormalities, preeclampsia, prematurity, stillbirth, and very large infants.[23]

In cases of gestational diabetes that are carefully controlled by doctors, however, the risks are fewer. For mothers, the most serious concern is increased frequency of preeclampsia. For infants, the major concern is macrosomia (an excessively large baby). This leads to long labors and difficult vaginal deliveries. There is an increased rate of cesarean section. Your baby, having become used to high blood glucose levels during pregnancy, produces high insulin levels and may suffer from very low blood sugar immediately after birth.

In the past, women whose gestational diabetes was very poorly controlled had an increased number of stillbirths, much like type 1 diabetics. However, several studies have demonstrated that good blood sugar control combined with careful fetal monitoring during the third trimester can reduce this risk to the same level as that of a normal population.[24]

The development of gestational diabetes, especially in the woman who is overweight, often predicts the development of type 2 diabetes later in life. A group of 603 gestational diabetics was followed for fifteen years after their deliveries.[25] Thirty-four percent of these women became diabetic after pregnancy.

The Management of the Diabetic Pregnancy

In overweight women who are at risk for gestational diabetes, ideal management should begin before conception with a screening test in order to unmask preexisting but undiagnosed type 2 diabetes. If this is found, good blood sugar control should be achieved before attempting pregnancy. This is because we know that very high blood sugar is associated with an increase in congenital abnormalities and miscarriage.

If preconceptual screens are normal, or have not been done, you should be screened in the first trimester and again in the second trimester. Once the diagnosis has been made, nutritional education and a diabetic diet should be instituted. The calorie recommendations must be individualized and depend upon body weight. The nutritional section of this book contains detailed diet plans for the overweight gestational diabetic.

For the majority of women, diet alone will be successful in maintaining normal blood sugars. Blood sugars can be monitored using a home glucose monitoring device. This usually involves pricking your finger to obtain a drop of blood, placing the blood on a test stick, and inserting it into a calibrated machine. A fasting glucose value, and tests before and either one or two hours after meals, will determine the degree of glucose control. The Fourth International Workshop Conference on Gestational Diabetes Mellitus recommended that blood sugar values should be less than 95 mg/ml before meals, less than 140 mg/ml at one hour after eating, and less than 120 mg/ml two hours after eating. A persistent fasting blood glucose value of greater than 95 mg/ml, after dietary therapy has been initiated, is an indication that insulin therapy is required.[26] Oral agents, the mainstay of therapy in type 2 diabetes, are not allowed in pregnancy because of their effects on the baby.

Physicians differ in how frequently they monitor their pregnant diabetic patients. Some test only fasting blood sugar every one to two weeks. Others require daily home checks both fasting and after eating. The frequency of monitoring depends on the severity of the diabetes and is usually done daily in women requiring insulin.

In addition to monitoring the mother's glucose values, fetal testing is normally initiated in the third trimester. The goal of glucose control is to minimize the chance of a very large baby and to eliminate the risk of diabetes-related stillbirth. The baby's status can be followed by a combination of ultrasound and fetal heart rate monitoring. Ultrasound can evaluate fetal weight, fetal breathing, movement, tone, and the amount of amniotic fluid. The Nonstress Test is a fetal heart-rate observation that looks at the response of the fetal heart to the baby's movements. A satisfactory Nonstress Test is an excellent predictor of a healthy baby.

A scoring system called the *Biophysical Profile* is a quantitative way of assessing your baby's well-being. Two points each are assigned for:

a satisfactory Nonstress Test

fetal breathing observed

fetal movement observed

fetus in a flexed position

adequate fluid

A score of 10 reflects a healthy baby. If the score is 6 or lower, we seriously consider delivery, or if the baby is premature, admission to the hospital with careful monitoring of baby and blood sugars until delivery can be safely accomplished.

Fetal macrosomia is usually defined as a baby estimated to

weigh 4,500 grams (10 pounds) or more. These babies are at high risk for shoulder dystocia, a situation in which the head delivers and the shoulders get stuck. This can be life threatening for both baby and mother, or can result in a broken arm, broken clavicle, or permanent neurological damage to the arm. Because of this risk, many obstetricians choose to deliver these very large babies by elective cesarean section rather than allowing a trial of labor. Those who do allow a labor trial will often choose not to use forceps or other instruments if the mother is unable to easily push the infant out.

Postpartum Caveats

Although gestational diabetes usually disappears immediately after delivery, if you have been diagnosed as suffering from it, it is wise to repeat your glucose screen six to eight weeks postpartum and to do it yearly thereafter. Diabetes in pregnancy is a warning sign that type 2 diabetes may follow.

Other Diagnostic Dilemmas

A very heavy abdomen makes diagnosis during pregnancy more difficult. The routine measurement of uterine height, from the pubic bone to the top of the uterus, is a good measure of fetal growth. The height in centimeters, in normal weight women, is usually equal to the number of weeks of gestation. In obese women, however, it is hard to distinguish what part of the measurement is mom and what part is baby, thereby increasing the risk of underestimating or overestimating fetal growth.

The accuracy of ultrasound measurements is decreased when this test is performed through a large fatty layer, which makes it more difficult to determine the baby's weight and status. It is harder to find the fetal heartbeat and to do an accurate Nonstress Test. It is also harder to obtain accurate blood pressure.

This chapter has discussed the problems that can develop in pregnant women who are overweight. Linda's story is an excellent illustration of these problems. In the two chapters that follow it, we will discuss labor, delivery, and postpartum complications.

Linda's Story

Linda first came to our office when she was twenty-three years old and newly married. At five foot one and over 200 pounds, it was clear that she had a problem with her weight. She had come in because she wanted to start a family and was having extremely irregular periods. She had also had two previous miscarriages. As a nurse, she was aware that the irregularity meant she was not ovulating and would need help conceiving. Two significant aspects of her medical history were a car accident with pelvic fractures at the age of six and hypertension, for which she had taken medication for a year. At the time of her first visit, her blood pressures were at the upper limit of normal. After an exam and an evaluation, which confirmed her self-diagnosis, she was started on the fertility drug Clomid. It was not easy to induce ovulation for Linda, and she required twice the usual dose of medication. Once she ovulated, however, she turned out to be quite fertile and became pregnant immediately.

Weight has always been a problem for me, ever since I graduated high school. Although my parents weren't overweight, I grew up eating lots of junk food and fast food. Being overweight in high school made me quite depressed, but it was very easy to lose weight when I was young. I started exercis-

ing, lived on granola bars and Dr Pepper, and lost 50 pounds. At that time I was 119, the thinnest I'd ever been. I kept it off for a few years, but by the time I met my husband, I was up to 140. We dated for a year, became engaged, and during the engagement I went to Weight Watchers. I was twenty-one when we got married and weighed 130 at our wedding.

I kept the weight off for a few months after the wedding, but when we were married six months I became pregnant and had a miscarriage. After that the weight just accumulated. I didn't exercise. We ate late and ate out a lot, fast food and junk food. I didn't know how to cook or even how to shop for groceries when I was first married. Before I became pregnant again, I tried to lose some weight. I went on one of those liquid diets and lost 25 pounds in two weeks, but it all came back very rapidly, and then some.

Linda began her first pregnancy at a weight of 221½ pounds at eight weeks gestation. Her blood pressure was slightly elevated at 146/88. She was sent for a nutritional consult with the aim of teaching her how to eat healthy foods during the pregnancy so that she would gain just enough weight, and not any extra. The possibility of starting her on an antihypertensive drug was considered, but knowing that blood pressure always drops in the second trimester of pregnancy, we opted to wait and see. By twenty weeks of gestation, Linda's weight was only 221 pounds. She was tested early for diabetes in pregnancy and had normal blood sugars. Her blood pressures remained normal throughout her second trimester.

I was concerned that my weight would cause problems for me. I'd heard about people gaining anywhere from 30 to 70 pounds during pregnancy, and I considered going to the Weight Watchers pregnancy diet program. As it turned out,

I was sick during all my pregnancy. I started throwing up before I even missed my period and threw up the morning of my cesarean section. Being nauseated all the time pretty much controlled my eating. I did worry about gaining too much weight, but mostly I was so happy to be having a baby that I figured I'd just deal with any weight gain afterward.

At twenty-eight weeks Linda had still gained no weight. At that point an ultrasound showed the baby to be too small. Linda was placed on bed rest with detailed instructions about food intake, and within another two weeks achieved appropriate fetal growth and a few pounds of weight gain.

At thirty-two weeks Linda was admitted in preterm labor with the symptoms of early toxemia of pregnancy, an elevated blood pressure of 142/78, and protein in her urine. The early labor was stopped, and she was sent home at bed rest with ultrasounds and fetal heart-rate tracings twice a week. Her blood pressure did not get worse on bed rest, but a week later she was admitted once again in early labor and her contractions were stopped. She continued at home with twice-weekly testing until thirty-eight weeks. At that time her weight was 235, a total pregnancy weight gain of 14 pounds, her blood pressure 150/100, and she was exhibiting increased reflexes. Her toxemia was clearly getting worse, her baby was mature, and it was time to deliver.

Because of Linda's childhood pelvic fractures, her pelvis was contracted, and a vaginal delivery was out of the question. Therefore she was admitted for a scheduled cesarean section, which proceeded smoothly. Linda gave birth to a healthy 6-pound 12-ounce baby girl.

My daughter's birth had scared me. I was frightened by the toxemia and by the fact that she might have been delivered prematurely. I breast-fed for a few months and then went back on the liquid diet and lost 60 pounds. That weight loss only lasted a few months, however, and then all the old habits reasserted themselves. I had a child, I was thrilled, and I was eating a lot but for different reasons. My husband and I really enjoyed our time together after she went to sleep. We ate our way through the evening—pizza and fast food in front of the television.

Four years later Linda conceived spontaneously but miscarried immediately. She tried again and was successful. This pregnancy began at age twenty-nine at an initial weight of 275 pounds. At ten weeks gestation, her first complication occurred, intractable nausea and vomiting requiring hospitalization and medication. Her blood pressures, in this pregnancy, were initially normal.

At twenty-eight weeks, weighing 281 pounds, she was admitted once again to rule out preterm labor. She was also screened for diabetes, and this time her blood sugar tests were grossly abnormal. Although many women with gestational diabetes can be managed on diet alone, Linda required insulin as well as a 2,000-calorie American Diabetes Association diet. As a nurse, Linda was very knowledgeable about diabetes, and comfortable giving herself insulin shots. She was also very careful with her diet and succeeded in maintaining good control over her blood sugar for the remainder of the pregnancy. At thirty-three weeks and 285 pounds, she began to develop the early signs of pregnancy-induced hypertension and was admitted to the hospital again for bed rest and stabilization. Her blood pressures initially came down, but just after thirty-five weeks were once again elevated and accompanied by headaches. At this time she underwent an amniocentesis to evaluate the baby for lung maturity. Babies of diabetic mothers often mature more slowly, and it was desirable, if possible, to deliver a baby with mature lungs. Fortunately the results of the amniocentesis were positive, and Linda, weighing 288 pounds, had a repeat cesarean section and tubal ligation at just under thirty-six weeks gestation. Her second baby was a healthy boy. Linda had gained only 13 pounds during this pregnancy.

During my second [successful] pregnancy I was very careful to keep my carbohydrates under control and not to eat anything with sugar. I saw a nutritionist regularly and also went to the diabetes clinic at the hospital every week. I was also nauseated during this whole pregnancy, which helped control my eating.

After my son was born, my weight had a lot of ups and downs. I went to Weight Watchers at one point and lost 96 pounds. Over the past eleven years, we've had a lot of stress in our family. Both my children are diabetic, and my husband became diabetic as well. I'm a borderline diabetic and can really tell the difference in my blood sugars depending on my weight. With all the medical problems in our family, I've responded to the stress by eating and gaining. Just recently, however, I had a real scare. We were taking a walk, and all of a sudden the left side of my face became numb. I thought to myself, "This is it. I'm not going to live to see my children graduate." At that point I weighed 304 pounds. I went back to Weight Watchers immediately and have lost 30 pounds in the past month. I've started exercising every day on my treadmill. We don't eat fast food or junk food any longer because I need to feed my diabetic family foods that are healthy for them. I've even taken some cooking classes so I can make interesting, healthy meals. Even so, it's easy to backslide and gain weight. It's a vicious circle. I get depressed. I eat too much. I gain weight and I get more depressed and eat even more. Sometimes I eat so much I can hardly move. On Weight Watchers I'm allowed only half the amount of food I was eating. I've come to terms with the fact that this kind of eating isn't just till I lose 50 pounds or 100 pounds. I'm going to have to eat like this forever.

Linda's case exhibits many of the pitfalls and problems encountered by the truly obese mother. These included elevated blood pressure, toxemia of pregnancy, diabetes, excessive weight gain in the postpartum period, miscarriage, preterm labor, and early delivery. It also illustrates a very typical pattern of cyclic weight loss followed by gaining even more weight. Fortunately, despite two extremely difficult pregnancies, Linda had two safe deliveries and two beautiful children. Her case illustrates the fact that significantly overweight mothers are at much higher risk and need careful follow-up by a knowledgeable obstetrician, nutritionist, and perinatologist.

Chapter Five

Delivery Plus

Complications of Labor and Birth

I n overweight and obese mothers, the labor and delivery process is subject to an increased rate of cesarean section, both primary and repeat, an increase in the need to induce or augment labor, higher blood loss, anesthesia difficulties, and infant complications usually related to very large size.

Cesarean Sections

Multiple factors contribute to the increased rate of cesarean section, which has been noted in many studies. If you are hypertensive, toxemic, or have gestational diabetes, you may have your labor induced because either you or your baby is deteriorating. At the time the induction becomes necessary, your cervix may not be ripe, and induction may be difficult to accomplish or may fail. In addition, if your baby is already compromised because of high blood pressure and decreased placental blood flow, he may not tolerate labor well and may show signs of distress during contractions. Obese mothers have larger babies than normal-weight mothers, and even when labor starts spontaneously, the large baby may not be able to navigate the birth canal. Even if you have a generous bony pelvis, excess fatty tissue in the vaginal passage may make it more difficult for an average-weight baby to pass. Finally, if you have gestational diabetes and a large baby, the baby is at risk for shoulder dystocia, a complication in which the head delivers vaginally and the shoulders become impacted. Rather than risk this complication, many obstetricians will choose to deliver a diabetic mother by cesarean section if her baby's weight estimate is over 4,000 grams.

There is considerable evidence in the medical literature showing that obese women have a higher cesarean section rate. Of 20,130 women who gave birth in New York State during a one-year period (1994–1995), women with a BMI over 29 were 1.64 times as likely to have a primary cesarean than were lower-weight women.[1]

Among 1,881 low-risk women who were delivered at a hospital-certified nurse midwifery practice, women with a BMI > 29 had a 7.7 percent cesarean-section rate compared with a 4.1 percent rate for women with BMI < 29.[2] A study of 887 high-parity Israeli women found a 19.6 percent cesarean rate in obese women versus 10.8 percent in the control group.[3] Although these are low rates, it was clear that the risk of cesarean was higher for obese women.

In massively obese women (> 300 pounds) the primary cesarean-section rate was 32.4 percent versus 14.3 percent in a normal-weight control group.[4] However, when women with diabetes and hypertension were excluded, there were no significant differences in outcome. This means that the increased risks were due to the medical complications that accompany obesity and not to the obesity itself. Another study of massively obese women reported a 31 percent cesarean section rate versus 8.6 percent for controls.[5]

A cesarean section is much more difficult to perform if you are obese and can lead to prolonged operating times and increased blood loss. The usual incision for cesarean is called a Pfannenstiel, nicknamed the "bikini cut." It is a transverse incision usually placed about two finger widths above your pubic bone. Usually this places the incision just at or below the vulvar hairline. If you are very heavy, your abdomen often hangs on or below the vulva, creating a warm, moist area that is susceptible to wound infection. Retracting the heavy abdomen to expose the area of the incision is a difficult job, often requiring an extra surgical assistant. Exposure of the underlying layers and the uterus is more difficult, and the heavy abdominal wall obstructs delivery of the fetal head. Thus, you might require a wider incision to deliver. Some surgeons prefer to use an up-and-down incision for cesareans in obese women, but this also has its problems. Although a long midline incision provides good exposure, there is more tension on the wound and this wound also is at risk for infection and coming apart.

There is evidence that in massively obese women, both the operating time and the blood loss are increased. One author found increased operative time in 48 percent of obese women versus 9.3 percent of controls and a blood loss of greater than one liter in 34.9 percent versus 9.3 percent of controls.[6] Another studied 1,610 women who had cesarean section, 127 of whom had a hemorrhage estimated at 1,500 ml or more.[7] Obesity of 250 pounds or above increased the odds of such a hemorrhage thirteen times. Given the increased risk associated with obesity, it is wise to be prepared for a potential transfusion. You can donate units of your own blood well in advance of delivery or can arrange for donors of your blood type to make blood available.

Complications of Anesthesia

Epidural anesthesia is the most common anesthesia for labor and cesarean section. A hollow needle is inserted into your back between two vertebrae and into the epidural space. This space is just outside the membrane, which covers the spinal cord. A thin catheter is threaded into the space, and local anesthetic is then placed. The catheter is left in so that additional medication may be delivered as needed. The epidural provides complete pain relief during labor and, with a larger amount of medication, gives complete anesthesia for cesarean section. In placing the needle, the distance from the skin surface to the epidural space varies with BMI.[8] The distance is shorter if you are in the sitting position than it is if you are lying on your side. Very heavy women may require an extra long needle even to reach the epidural space. In a comparison of 117 massively obese women with controls, 42 percent of the obese group but only 6 percent of the controls required multiple tries for successful placement of the epidural catheter.[9] For those women who required a general anesthetic, placement of the endotracheal tube was difficult in 35 percent of obese women and in none of the controls. Multiple failures have been reported in epidural placement in obese women.[10]

Maternal Obesity and Its Consequences for the Baby

As we have pointed out in prior chapters, obese mothers are more likely to have very large babies, regardless of the amount of gestational weight gain. This is particularly true of women with gestational diabetes. Obstetricians use the term *fetal macrosomia* to describe babies whose birthweight is 4,500 grams or above. Thirty percent of babies in one study of massively obese women were macrosomic, and another study had a 16 percent rate of macrosomia in obese mothers versus 8 percent for normal controls.[11, 12]

Several factors contribute to an exceptionally large baby. The parents may be genetically very large individuals. The mother may be obese or diabetic. A previous very large baby suggests that the next one may be equally large, and babies who are overdue are bigger. Macrosomic babies have wide shoulders and heads that are harder and less likely to mold as they pass through the birth canal.

One possible outcome is simply an arrest of labor. Your cervix dilates up to a point and then quits because your baby's head is unable to descend farther. Another scenario is that your cervix dilates completely, but you are unable to push the infant out because the head is stuck. In these cases, a cesarean is performed.

The most dangerous outcome is shoulder dystocia. In this situation, you push out the head, but the shoulders get stuck in back of the pubic bone. A number of obstetrical maneuvers can be done to help the delivery. Usually your legs are pulled way up and back to open your pelvis. A huge episiotomy is performed, often cutting into the rectum. This provides additional room. The baby is then rotated so that its shoulders are in the diagonal of the pelvis and an attempt is made to deliver the posterior arm. While these maneuvers are usually successful, they can have serious consequences for both you and your child. You may have a huge episiotomy and major blood loss. The baby can have a broken arm or broken clavicle. There can be neurological damage to the nerves that supply the arm, a condition called Erb's palsy. This may or may not resolve spontaneously. Even worse, the baby can suffer brain damage from oxygen deprivation if the delivery takes a long time. If the body cannot be delivered, the outcome is infant death. Birth mortality is almost double for infants over 4,500 grams as a result of birth trauma associated with difficult delivery.[13]

Babies weighing 4,000 grams or more constitute about 5 percent of all deliveries in the United States. Babies weighing over 4,500 grams are .4 percent.[14] Considering the millions of children born every year, even these small percentages constitute large numbers. It would be ideal if we could predict the difficult delivery ahead of time and then perform a cesarean section in order to avoid trauma. Unfortunately, the use of ultrasound to estimate fetal weight does not always yield accurate results, and this is especially so in the obese woman. Even if it were possible to predict fetal weight with complete accuracy, many women are perfectly capable of delivering large babies vaginally without difficulty. In 1991, at Parkland Hospital in Texas, 99.5 percent of babies weighing between 4,000 to 4,500 grams who were delivered vaginally did not suffer any complications. This was also true of 96.6 percent of babies over 4,500 grams.[15] Thus, if we were to perform cesarean sections on all women whose babies were estimated to weigh over 4,000 grams, we would be performing many unnecessary operations. At the present time it is impossible to accurately predict which deliveries will result in shoulder dystocia.

There are, however, certain factors that should make an obstetrician suspicious and cautious. We know that women who are obese, diabetic, and post term are more likely to have very large babies. Labors that require an excessively long time to push out the fetal head, labors in which the contractions become ineffective and which require Pitocin to continue, and deliveries that require the aid of instruments appear to be associated with a higher risk of shoulder dystocia. Thus a prudent obstetrician might wish to deliver a high-risk woman a week or two early, and avoid prolonged pushing and midpelvis operative maneuvers.

In the next chapter we will examine postpartum complications and look at the impact of obesity on recovery.

Chapter Six

Big, Beautiful plus Baby

Complications in the Postpartum Period

Although the vast majority of overweight mothers will have an uneventful recovery from childbirth, a number of complications are significantly increased in women who are very obese. These include wound infections, wound separations, uterine infection, and venous blood clots, all of which can lead to a prolonged hospital stay.

Wound Problems

As we have already pointed out, if you are overweight, you are more likely to have a cesarean section; thus more overweight women have abdominal incisions to begin with. Wound infections and the separation of the incision even without an infection are common complications. A thick layer of abdominal fat allows fluid to accumulate. This fluid comes from leakage, through the capillaries, of the serum in which blood cells float. The accumulated fluid is called a *seroma*. The seroma will spread the wound apart, and eventually, because the fluid needs to drain, will force a hole to develop in the skin layer of the incision. If bacteria invade the space as well, white blood cells will migrate to the wound and pus will form. The skin usually becomes red and painful. The infection, much like a pimple, will eventually force itself to the surface and begin to drain.

When these complications develop, and your physician recognizes them early, he will usually open the wound and probe it with a Q-tip to allow the fluid or pus to drain. Your wound is then washed several times a day with hydrogen peroxide solution, and antibiotics are started. As long as the wound is kept clean and allowed to drain, the tissue will heal in from below, and eventually the incision will close. Most of the time your scar is no wider than it would have been had there been no problem.

How often do these complications take place? Among 2,431 women who had cesareans during a one-year period 2.8 percent developed wound infections and 1.7 percent developed seromas.[1] Morbid obesity made it more likely that a wound infection would take place. Other factors increasing the risk were an emergency delivery and rupture of membranes for more than six hours. There appears to be a strong correlation between maternal weight and the development of a wound infection with as much as an 8.4-fold increase in wound infections among obese women.[2, 3] One surgeon looked at whether suturing the fatty layer closed decreased the risk of seromas and infections. He studied 245 women who had a fatty layer at least 2 cm thick. In half the women, the layer was closed. In the other half, only the skin was closed. Women in whom the fatty layer was closed had a 14 percent rate of infections and seromas, compared with 26 percent for the women whose fatty layer was not closed.[4] Thus, surgical technique, as well as weight, influences a woman's risk of this particular set of complications.

Uterine Infections

A postpartum uterine infection called *endometritis* can occur with or without a cesarean section. The uterine lining (the endometrium) becomes contaminated by bacteria, most often from the vagina. In the preantibiotic era, endometritis was a major cause of maternal death. Uterine infection often accompanies excessively long labors in which the membranes have been ruptured for many hours. This allows bacteria plenty of time to work their way upward in the reproductive tract.

These infections always cause fever and can be promptly diagnosed and treated with intravenous antibiotics. During cesarean section, a prophylactic dose of antibiotics is usually given to prevent endometritis. Several authors have reported an increased risk for obese women: a 45 percent incidence of endometritis versus 0 percent for nonobese women.[5, 6, 7] Although both uterine and wound infections can be easily treated, they can result in a longer hospital stay.

Blood Clots

Pregnancy, in general, is a time of increased risk for blood clots in the leg veins. Clotting is a complex mechanism, involving multiple proteins produced in the liver. During pregnancy, two factors contribute to the increased risk of clots. High estrogen levels cause the liver to synthesize more clotting proteins. A heavy uterus puts pressure on the vena cava, the large vein that brings blood back to the heart from the legs. This slows the blood flow and increases the chance that a clot may form.

After delivery, the injury caused by the birth releases substances into the blood that trigger clotting. Ideally this should only stop bleeding from vessels that have been severed by trauma or by a deliberate cesarean or episiotomy incision. However, if you are bedridden for several days and do not move around, your chances of developing a blood clot in your leg are increased. This often happens if you have had a cesarean section and are in pain. Being very obese makes it more difficult to maneuver, and you may be less likely to make the effort to walk around soon after surgery. Special stockings called Ted Hose are often prescribed after cesarean. These elastic stockings help compress the veins and increase blood flow. A more sophisticated device called the SCD (sequential compression device) is a cuff that is wrapped around your legs from ankle to thigh and that inflates and deflates to move blood along. Both Ted Hose and SCDs help avoid undesirable clotting.

The most dangerous blood complication is called a *pulmonary embolism*. This happens when a piece of clot from your leg breaks off and is carried to your lung. A clot in the lung causes breathing difficulties; if unrecognized and untreated, it can be fatal.

Once again, although these complications are rare, they can occur more frequently in very heavy women.[8] The risks can be minimized by the use of stockings and SCDs and by walking after delivery, as soon as possible and as much as possible.

Evaluating Your Risks of Complications

Although the overall trend certainly supports increasing risk with increasing weight, it is important to distinguish between overweight, obese, and morbidly obese. Many of the studies that we have cited apply primarily to what are called "morbidly obese" women. Whereas there is general agreement in the medical community that a BMI above 30 is obese, authors have used different definitions for morbidly obese. These have included BMI > 35, BMI > 40, or weight > 250 pounds. Most women who are merely overweight can expect to have an uncomplicated course. The heavier you are, however, the more alert and knowledgeable you need to be.

The second half of this book will focus on nutrition and help you establish healthy eating patterns for your pregnancy and beyond.

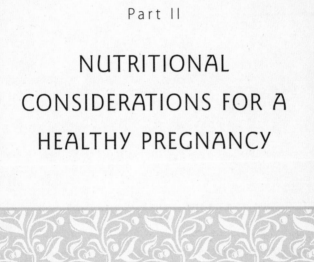

Part II

NUTRITIONAL CONSIDERATIONS FOR A HEALTHY PREGNANCY

Chapter Seven

Dietitians' Details

For most women, eating during pregnancy can be a very enjoyable experience. For the plus-size woman, however, eating properly at this time can be one of the greatest challenges of her life. She should consider her pregnancy as an opportunity to make behavioral changes that can ultimately improve her health and, more importantly, the well-being of her baby. The following chapters will describe what is necessary to eat before, during, and after pregnancy to ensure a healthy outcome for mother and baby, both physically and emotionally.

As you learned in earlier chapters, there are many factors that contribute to your weight. As a result, what you weigh is not always your choice. We assume that if you are reading this book, you are overweight and pregnant or trying to get pregnant. As with all new moms, your main concern is to have a healthy pregnancy and deliver a healthy baby. Learning to eat healthier will benefit not only you but your family as well, no matter what you weigh.

We hope that the chapters in this section will provide some healthy tips about eating and help you gain the appropriate amount of weight during your pregnancy.

What Our Patients Tell Us

Here is a partial list of the things our patients have taught us about themselves over the years.

- Some people don't know what's healthy to eat.

- Some people say, "No one ever taught me how to eat right."

- Some people know what to eat but can't control what they eat.

- Most people enjoy eating.

- Some people think about food all the time.

- When it comes to pregnancy, *all* women want a healthy baby.

Any or all of these might be true for you. The truth is, food choices and weight management can be complicated. We hope the information we provide will help you take control of your eating.

Before the Food "Talk"

Before we address the nutrition issues, here are some tips that our clients have incorporated into their lives. Though many were unsuccessful in controlling their weight before pregnancy, these tips were nevertheless useful because they helped take our patients' focus off food. Little by little, they realized that small changes significantly improved their eating habits and overall health.

Check them off as you incorporate them into your life.

☐ Eat slowly; put your fork down in between bites.

☐ Recognize signs of feeling full and stop eating when you feel them.

☐ Never eat while reading or watching TV.

☐ When out for a meal, split larger entrées with a friend or take home the extra for another meal.

☐ Order an appetizer as a main dish (after soup or salad).

☐ Always ask for dressings, sauces, and spreads on the side.

☐ Drink plenty of water with your meal.

☐ Resist the urge to go on fad diets that promise quick weight loss. Remember, if those diets were so great, everyone would be thin.

☐ Take advantage of friends and family who will support you in your quest for a healthy future. Stay away from people who want to sabotage your efforts to change your eating and life habits.

☐ Give up the excuses! Schedule special events in your life and plan ahead. If you feel like eating a little more one day, be sure you compensate the following day.

☐ Visit the Web sites of your favorite fast-food restaurants to help you with your food selections when you eat at them. Every large restaurant chain now posts nutrition information on the Web or has it available at the restaurant.

As a new mom, you want to impart healthy eating behaviors to, and set a good example for, your family. Remember, your children will learn by your actions rather than by your words. They will look to you as a role model and imitate your habits. Getting children off to a good start with food choices may help prevent them from "carrying a little extra" as they grow older.

What You Can Do Before You Get Pregnant

If you are already pregnant, you may skip to chapter 8, which focuses on nutrition requirements during pregnancy. If you are not, read the next few paragraphs to help prepare yourself nutritionally for becoming pregnant.

Being in a good nutritional state before you get pregnant is as important as your nutritional state during pregnancy. This is why we recommend that you start eating a well-balanced diet when you first decide that you want to become a parent. The most well-known nutrition guideline for eating healthily is the Food Guide Pyramid. It contains all of the food groups and gives the proper number of daily servings in each group. The pyramid shape visually displays the foods so that you can see what groups you should eat and in what quantities. The top section contains foods that are to be used in smaller quantities. As

Food Pyramid
Figure 1

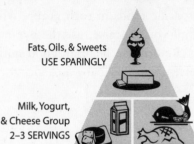

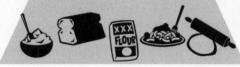

Fats, Oils, & Sweets
USE SPARINGLY

Milk, Yogurt,
& Cheese Group
2–3 SERVINGS

Meat, Poultry, Fish, Dry Beans,
Eggs & Nuts Group
2–3 SERVINGS

Vegetable Group
3–5 SERVINGS

Fruit Group
2–4 SERVINGS

Bread, Cereal, Rice,
& Pasta Group
6–11 SERVINGS

Source: Food and Nutrition Information Center of the National Agriculture Library of the U.S. Department of Agriculture

How to Use the Daily Food Guide
What counts as one serving?

Breads, Cereals, Rice, and Pasta
1 slice of bread
1/2 cup of cooked rice or pasta
1/2 cup of cooked cereal
1 ounce of ready-to eat cereal

Vegetables
1/2 cup of chopped raw or cooked vegetables
1 cup of leafy raw vegetables

Fruits
1 piece of fruit or melon wedge
3/4 cup of juice
1/2 cup of canned fruit
1/4 cup of dried fruit

Milk, Yogurt, and Cheese
1 cup of milk or yogurt
1 1/2 to 2 ounces of cheese

**Meats, Poultry, Fish, Dry Beans,
Eggs, and Nuts**
2 1/2 to 3 ounces of cooked lean meat, poultry,
   or fish
Count 1/2 cup of cooked beans, or 1 egg, or
   2 tablespoons of peanut butter as 1 ounce
   of lean meat (about 1/3 serving)

Fats, Oils, Sweets
LIMIT CALORIES FROM THESE

you go down the levels, the sections get bigger, indicating that you can eat more of these foods. When you get to chapter 9, you will learn about more specific foods in each group, which we refer to as "blocks." Until you conceive, use the pyramid as a basis for healthy eating. Remember, being in good nutritional health before you conceive gives your baby a chance for a very healthy start.

Chapter Eight

Dining in Utero

How Much Can I Gain?

Most pregnant women are surprised to find out the concept of eating for two is really not true. What the literature recommends is an additional 300 calories per day to a well-balanced diet beginning in the second trimester. Caloric requirements are quite individualized based on what a woman was eating at the time of conception. Eating for two does not mean eating double what you usually eat.

Pregnant women, large or small, usually start off by asking the same question: "How much weight can I gain?" The answer is based on looking at many factors, including your height, weight, age, activity level, rate of weight gain, and history of prior pregnancies. Generally, if you are a plus-size mom, you need to gain about one-half to three-quarters of a pound per week (approximately two to three pounds per month). Most women gain less in the early part of their pregnancy and more in the last months. The question is how are you going to get there?

According to the recommendations we wrote in Section I of this book, plus-size women should not gain less than 15 pounds and not more than 25 pounds. Quite often pregnant women become motivated to eat properly for the first time in their lives when they feel the responsibility for another human being. We discourage them from turning this time into a weight-loss diet and encourage them to use it as a time to begin good eating habits. The pattern of weight gain should be gradual and steady.

Calorie Requirements

In terms of exact calories, should all pregnant women eat an additional 300 calories no matter what they weigh? The answer is that each case is very different. You will need to ask your doctor what the weight-gain goal is for you. Calorie levels will be based on many factors and will most likely be adjusted as your pregnancy progresses. In the case of multiple births, the goal is an additional 10 pounds for twins and generally 5 to 10 pounds for each additional baby. More important than the exact number of calories is achieving a slow, steady weight gain by eating a well-balanced diet. Chapter 9 will give you many examples of a well-balanced diet for pregnancy.

The Nutrients for a Healthy Diet

CARBOHYDRATES

Carbohydrates, often referred to as "carbs," should be the main source of energy (calories) in your diet. Carbs contribute important vitamins, minerals, and fiber, and some carbohydrate foods even contain protein. All of these are necessary to a healthy eating plan. Carbs are divided into two groups: complex and simple. Complex carbs include starches, beans, potatoes, rice, cereals, corn, and vegetables. Simple carbs include fruits, juices, candy, sugar, and honey. Selecting carbs that are high in fiber can help keep you full, prevent constipation, and keep your blood sugar under control. For the plus-size pregnancy, having a whole-grain waffle topped with fresh berries is a better choice than a refined-white-flour waffle topped with butter and syrup. This might require retraining your taste buds, but in the end, both you and your baby will benefit. Many carbohydrate ideas will be listed for you in the meal planning section in chapter 9.

PROTEIN

Protein is commonly called the "building block" of life because it helps create the cells and tissues of the fetus. Most pregnant women are already eating adequate amounts of protein. The recommended dietary allowance of protein is 60 grams per day during pregnancy. This translates into eating at least six ounces of animal protein per day (chicken, fish, beef, and eggs) and 2.5 glasses of milk. That is the bare minimum. Most women are eating more because there is also protein in breads, pasta, cereals, beans, and vegetables. Therefore, it's not difficult to meet the basic protein goal. Overall, protein should represent about 20 to 25 percent of your total calorie intake. Lacto-ovo vegetarians have no problem meeting this goal by including eggs, cheese, and milk in their diet. However, vegans, who do not include any protein from animal sources, need to consult with a registered dietitian for specific meal planning. In the case of the plus-size pregnancy, choosing lean meats and low-fat dairy products is the best way to meet the protein goal without extra calories and fat. An ounce of grilled or poached fish will give you the same protein as an ounce of fried fish but with half the calories and a lot less fat.

FATS

Fats are an additional source of energy in your diet and provide calories for the growing fetus. This is not the time to be fat free but also not the time for the "Friday fried fish special." Fats should be of good quality, such as that found in nuts and avocados rather than in shortening, lard, and hydrogenated and saturated fats. Putting a few slices of avocado into your turkey sandwich is a better choice than eating guacamole dip and high-fat chips. Fats should represent approximately 30 percent of your total calorie intake, although it is inevitable that on some days it may be higher or lower than others.

FLUIDS

Whether or not you are pregnant, fluids are an essential part of a healthy meal plan. An average goal for fluid intake should be eight glasses per day. If it's a hot summer day, you may need more, just as you would if you were engaging in a high level of exercise. Not having enough fluid may cause dehydration and preterm labor. This is what happened to one of the authors. While driving home from a dietitian's convention, Marlene did not drink much fluid for fear she might need too many bathroom breaks. As a result, she became dehydrated. When she arrived home, she didn't realize that the "strange" abdominal movement she was having was actually preterm labor. A quick trip to the hospital that night was the beginning of her bed-rest period for the next three months. Because of stories like this, we recommend that when you are thirsty, you drink to satisfy your thirst.

Most plus-size women find that they can reduce the number of calories in their diet without having to change many food choices by replacing juices, regular sodas, and regular milk with water and nonfat milk. This is the perfect time to stop chugging down those high-calorie, high-sugar drinks. Do you know that 12 ounces of juice contain 9 teaspoons of sugar? This is the same amount as in one can of soda. Juice is often thought of as a healthy food because it's from fruit, but eating a whole piece of fruit will give you fewer calories, lots of fiber, and more vitamins and minerals as well as the same fluid as a half cup of juice.

VITAMINS AND MINERALS

Almost all of our patients take a prenatal vitamin/mineral supplement as recommended by their doctor. Quite often, these supplements are started prior to the pregnancy to ensure good nutritional status. This is particularly important in regard to folic acid. Vitamins are not a substitute for healthy food; they are an insurance policy to make sure your diet contains all essential vitamins and minerals. It is important to take the proper dose. Taking two pills is not better than taking one since an excess of vitamins at this time can be dangerous. Prenatal vitamins are especially high in folic acid and iron, which are needed in greater quantities during pregnancy. Folic acid intake prior to and throughout the pregnancy is important for the prevention of neural-tube defects such as spina bifida and anencephaly. Some of the best food sources of folic acid are fresh, uncooked fruits, leafy green vegetables, broccoli, spinach, brussels sprouts, oranges, beans, and fortified breads and cereals.

The American Dietetic Association recommends that adult pregnant women have a minimum of 1000 mg of calcium per day to help preserve their bones and teeth as well as the growing bones and teeth of their babies. Most doctors recommend between 1200–1500 mg of calcium per day from food sources or supplements. If your baby isn't getting enough calcium from your diet, your bones and teeth will suffer because you will be giving up calcium for your fetus. For those of you who can't drink milk and eat cheese, for whatever reason, calcium pills should be substituted.

Best Calcium Sources	Serving Size	Calcium (mg)
Low-fat or nonfat yogurt	8 ounces	300
1% or nonfat milk	8 ounces	300
Low-fat hard cheese	1 ounce	200
Broccoli (cooked)	½ cup	85
Almonds	1 ounce	75
Soybeans	½ cup	65
Low-fat cottage cheese	½ cup	65
Whole orange	1 medium	50

It is important to note that vitamin pills have no calories and will not affect your weight gain. Also important is the time when you take your supplements. An easy rule of thumb is to take your prenatal vitamin with your calcium at the end of a meal. If you are nauseated in the morning, take it with lunch or dinner. If you are also on an iron supplement, take it between meals with water. Eating a high-vitamin-C fruit such as an orange or grapefruit at this time will enhance your body's absorption of the iron.

NONNUTRITIVE SUBSTANCES

Nonnutritive substances such as artificial sweeteners may or may not be okay. Why take the risk? Most pregnant women agree to stop using these substances when we recommend it. Again, the long-term effects are not known, and given the fact that sugar contains only 16 calories per teaspoon, if it is used in moderation, it can be worked into a well-balanced diet. If you are diabetic or develop gestational diabetes, it may be necessary to use some of these products in moderation, but use them only with the consent of your doctor. If you do find it necessary to use an artificial sweetener, choose aspartame or Splenda because they are thought to be safer than saccharine.

ALCOHOL AND CAFFEINE

What would you think if you saw someone feeding an infant a gin and tonic or an espresso? You might feel they were abusing the baby. Well, it's no different when the fetus is in utero. Is it okay to have an occasional drink of alcohol? We really don't know because safe levels of alcohol consumption have not been established. When nutritionists are asked, we always recommend that the patient check with her doctor. Why not give your baby a great start by not consuming foods that are controversial? We feel that alcohol adds calories and weight to your body, and it can be detrimental to your child. It has been shown to be a contributing factor in birth defects, low birth weight, and additional complications. Since weight gain is of great concern, drinking alcohol at this time is strongly discouraged. If relaxation is a concern, try yoga, massage, or listen to some great music.

Caffeine is another substance that we discourage women from drinking during pregnancy. We've been told that it takes twice as long to leave the fetus as it does you. If it makes your heartbeat rapidly, think about how it affects your baby. Since not enough is known about the effects of caffeine on the unborn fetus, we encourage our patients to taper off their caffeine intake and then get off it altogether during their pregnancy. If you are not pregnant, take the time to wean yourself off of coffee, tea (hot or iced), cola, and chocolate. If these beverages contain sugar, you will save on empty calories. A suggestion to wean you off coffee is to start by mixing half-decaffeinated and half-regular coffee. You may also want to add more nonfat milk if it's hot or ice cubes if it's cold. A good rule of thumb is to have a maximum amount of 200 mg of caffeine per day.

If you're a person who consumes a lot of caffeine, you might feel a withdrawal effect. The way to handle these feelings is to eat every few hours and focus on healthy foods. Among the benefits of reducing caffeine is that you'll sleep better. You'll appreciate the extra sleep now because you're going to be losing it later! The caffeine content of each item on the following chart will depend on the brand you select. Most products list a toll-free phone number on the can or bottle which you can call to get specific caffeine information. Even though many decaffeinated coffee beverages have zero milligrams of caffeine, you still need to be aware of the empty calories they contain. It's best to drink water and low-calorie beverages and save your calories for foods that contain important nutrients.

Caffeine Chart

Food	Serving size	Caffeine (approximate)
Brewed coffee	8 ounces	137 mg
Instant coffee	1 teaspoon	57 mg
Instant coffee, decaf	1 teaspoon	2 mg
Cocoa or hot chocolate	8 ounces	5 mg
Tea, leaf or bag	8 ounces	36–50 mg
Flavored iced teas	8 ounces	15–24 mg
Green tea	8 ounces	30 mg
Herbal teas	8 ounces	0 mg
Diet cola	8 ounces	30–45 mg
Cola	8 ounces	30–45 mg
Root beer (reg. or diet)	8 ounces	0–14 mg
Orange soda	8 ounces	0–28 mg
Dr Pepper (reg. or diet)	8 ounces	28 mg
Lemon-lime (reg. or diet)	8 ounces	0 mg
Caffeine-free cola	8 ounces	0 mg
Coffee frozen yogurt	1 cup	40–80 mg
Coffee ice cream	1 cup	30–60 mg
Coffee yogurt (nonfrozen)	8 ounces	0–45 mg
Dark chocolate bar	1 ounce	20 mg
Milk chocolate bar	1 ounce	6 mg

Chapter Nine

Building the Baby, One Block at a Time

I n setting up a nutrition plan, the most important thing is to incorporate your best eating habits. This will be an "insurance policy" to help you survive this pregnancy and build a healthy baby. As we discuss each building block of nutrition, please refer to the lists in the "food blocks" that appear throughout this chapter. There you will find many meal-plan options. In each food category, when applicable, we will have up to three blocks or groupings of food. The foods listed in the A block are what we feel are the best choices because they give you the greatest nutrients or bulk for the fewest calories. The B and C blocks should be used in moderation.

The Milk / Yogurt Blocks

Calcium and protein are the most important nutrients in these building blocks. It is best to choose nonfat milk and yogurt products in the A-block because they contain the same calcium and protein as the B- and C-block choices but have fewer calories. For example, eight ounces of nonfat milk in the A block will have 300 mg of calcium and eight grams of protein, the same as in whole, regular milk in the C block. The regular milk contains an additional 90 calories of fat, which is equivalent to two pats of butter. Personally, we would rather save the butter for our toast than having it homogenized into the milk.

The A-block milk and yogurt foods are composed of nonfat milk and yogurt products. They get calories from the carbohydrate called lactose (milk sugar) and protein.

- 8 oz nonfat milk
- 8 oz nonfat yogurt
- ⅓ cup of nonfat dry milk
- 8 oz of 1 percent milk

The B-block milk and yogurt foods are also good choices but have more calories. If you choose foods with aspartame, they will contain similar calories to those foods in the A-block. As you read in chapter 8, we suggest that you limit your servings of aspartame to three or fewer per day.

- ½ cup nonfat or low-fat frozen yogurt
- 8 oz reduced-fat milk
- 8 oz low-fat yogurt
- 8 oz low-fat buttermilk

The C-block milk and yogurt foods are the least desirable to include as part of your diet. If you do select from this group, do it less often. Remember that there will be more calories for the same nutritional value.

- 8 oz whole milk
- 8 oz whole milk yogurt

The Meat Blocks

The meat blocks consist of poultry, beef, fish, cheese, tofu, beans, and other major protein sources in your diet. Protein is the main reason you need to choose foods in this group. You will get the same amount of protein whether you choose foods in the A, B, or C blocks. Again, the only difference is the amount of fat and calories. This is the time to get used to tasting the less greasy, fatty meats. A chicken breast without skin is an A-block meat. With skin, it moves to the B block, and if it's fried, it moves to the C block. The choice is yours. The more A-block choices you make, the healthier your diet. A sampling of A-block meats are listed below. Foods in this block should be prepared without adding fat. Instead of *f*rying your chicken, you can *b*ake, *b*roil, *b*oil, or *b*arbecue. As you can see, the B words are better than the F word "fried." It's interesting to note that sautéing, when it is done with oil or other types of fat, is the French word for frying.

- 1 oz skinless chicken breast
- 2 egg whites
- ¼ cup nonfat or low-fat cottage cheese
- 1 oz fish or shellfish
- 1 oz fat-free cheese

The B-block meats are also good choices but contain a little more fat than the choices in the A block.

- 1 oz chicken (with skin)
- 1 oz filet mignon
- 1 egg
- ¼ cup regular cottage cheese
- 4 oz tofu
- 1 oz string cheese

Once again, the C-block meat choices are the least desirable. If you do select from this group, watch your portion sizes and complement your meal with A and B blocks from the other food groups. For example, when you feel like you must have that piece of fried chicken, complement your meal with steamed vegetables and brown rice instead of mashed potatoes with gravy and creamed spinach.

- 1 oz fried chicken
- 1 oz cheddar cheese
- 1 oz spare ribs
- 1 oz pork sausage
- 1 oz prime rib

The Fruit Blocks

Fruits are carbohydrates that provide vitamins, minerals, and fiber. All fruits in their natural form fit into the A block. A small sample of fruits are listed below in proper portion sizes; the expanded list can be found at the end of this chapter. Finish each meal with a piece of fruit to help satisfy your sweet tooth. By doing this, you will surely crave fewer sweets.

- 1 apple
- ½ banana
- 1 cup melon
- 17 small grapes
- 12 cherries

The B-block fruits are also a good choice. Note, however, that dried fruits need to be measured carefully. Many people have a tendency to keep going back to the jar without measuring the amount of apricot halves, raisins, or dried cherries they're consuming. These foods are also a great way to naturally sweeten your cereal at breakfast.

- dried fruit that equals about 60 calories (read labels)
- 2 tablespoons raisins
- 8 apricot halves
- 3 dried prunes
- 1.5 large figs

Fruit juices are listed in the C-block fruits because they usually contain little to no fiber. Most people are unaware of the amount of calories in fruit juice. If you drink 12 oz of juice, the calories are identical to 12 oz of soda. What do you think would fill you up more—4 ounces of orange juice or a whole peeled orange? They both have the same numbers of calories, but the whole orange has approximately 3 grams of fiber. Remember, *fiber = full*. It will keep you feeling fuller longer. Unless you agree to use a measuring cup, take our advice and don't plan to drink too much juice during your pregnancy. Notice that mixed fruit beverages and smoothies are not included in these blocks. They are discussed in detail in chapter 13. Most people think such drinks are healthy, but do not realize how they pack in the calories.

- ½ cup apple juice
- ⅓ cup cranberry juice
- ⅓ cup grape juice
- ⅓ cup prune juice

The Vegetable Block

Good news! All foods in this group fit into the A-block. You can enjoy eating all the vegetables that you want as long as you are not adding fat to them. Remember that starchy vegetables such as beans, peas, corn, potatoes, and soybeans are part of the starch block.

- Raw vegetables
- Steamed vegetables
- Vegetable juice
- Steamed artichoke
- Vegetarian vegetable soup

The Starch Blocks

Starches are members of the expanded carbohydrate family. They provide you with energy and fiber. You will learn more about fiber in chapter 12. In the plans we have designed, you will be surprised to see that there will be plenty of starches to give you energy and keep your bowels running smoothly.

The A starch block contains foods that are usually high in fiber and low in fat. Below are a few examples. The more you choose starches from this block, the fuller you'll feel.

- 1 slice whole-wheat bread
- ½ cup beans

- ⅓ cup brown rice
- ½ cup whole-grain cereal
- 4–6 high-fiber crackers
- ½ cup yams
- 1 corn tortilla

The B starch blocks have little or no fat. That's the positive part. However, the negative side is that the foods are relatively low in fiber. Here are a few foods that belong to this block.

- 1 slice white bread
- ⅓ cup white rice
- 6 saltines
- ¾ cup Rice Krispies
- ½ cup mashed potatoes
- 1 flour tortilla

The C starch choices are the least desirable. In addition to containing complex carbohydrates, these starches are high in added fat, low in fiber, and may contain sugar. You should not be visiting this block too often. If you want to have a limited amount of french fries, have them with grilled chicken rather than fried chicken. Remember to round out the meal with steamed vegetables and fruit for dessert. Always plan to share your order of fries or ask for half an order only. Most restaurants will happily take your money for a full order and give you only a half order. Always try to ask yourself if you would rather have half the fries on you or out with the garbage. It's much easier to throw out the garbage than to "throw" the fat off your hips.

- Croissant
- French fries
- Biscuit
- Cookies

The Fat Building Blocks

Even if you choose all the fats in your diet from the A fat group, this does not mean that you can eat an unlimited quantity. All blocks are equal in calories in this food group. For example, one teaspoon of butter in the C-block is high in saturated fat and cholesterol but has the same calories as one-eighth of an avocado in the A block. The avocado is high monounsaturated fat, which is a "good" fat. Each choice has 45 calories.

The A-fat-block foods are usually high in monounsaturated fats. Many nuts and oils fit into this group. Below are a few examples.

- ⅛ avocado
- 1 teaspoon olive or canola oil
- 2 tablespoons low-fat salad dressing
- 2 teaspoons peanut butter
- 8–10 olives

The B-fat-block foods are almost as good a choice. This group is made up mainly of polyunsaturated fats. Below are a few examples.

- 1 tablespoon light mayonnaise
- 1 teaspoon corn or safflower oil
- 1 tablespoon salad dressing
- 1 tablespoon lower-fat margarine
- 1 tablespoon sunflower seeds

The C-fat-block foods are the least desirable. If you select from this group, do so less often and with caution. These fats are saturated and may not be as healthy for your heart as unsaturated fats. Below are a few examples.

- 3 tablespoons reduced-fat sour cream
- 1 tablespoon reduced-fat butter
- 2 slices turkey bacon
- 2 tablespoons light cream cheese

The "Free" Blocks

Free blocks include foods that are not "charged" to any block. You can choose these foods as often as you like to enhance your meals. Some items contain added salt. If your doctor tells you to watch your sodium intake, use these with caution. Foods higher in sodium are indicated with an asterisk.

- Herbs and spices
- Lemon and lime juice
- Fat-free salad dressings*
- Nonfat mayonnaise*
- Pickles*
- Nonstick cooking sprays

Note for Vegetarians

If you avoid meat but eat dairy products such as milk, cheese, and eggs, you are a lacto-ovo vegetarian. If you are eating a well-balanced diet, it will be possible for you to include the nutrients you need for building your baby. Simply select the foods you like from each food group. Note that cheese and eggs are in the meat group.

If you are a vegan, it is strongly recommended that you consult with a registered dietitian. It is difficult to meet all of the requirements for a pregnancy on a vegan diet. Often, when our vegan patients find out that they are pregnant, they agree to add some animal protein to their diet. Whether it is because they crave it or they feel the growing fetus needs it, they do this as a temporary measure. This added protein is like a security "baby" blanket to some women, by providing them with peace of mind. Vegan diets are of the greatest concern since they do not provide adequate amounts of vitamin B_{12}. Consult with your doctor regarding supplementation of this vitamin. In addition, vegan diets are often inadequate in calcium, iron, vitamin D, and zinc. In all of our years of counseling patients, we have never encountered a strictly vegan pregnant woman! If you choose not to add animal protein, complete proteins can be carefully made by combining foods such as beans with rice or peanut butter with whole-wheat bread. These combinations make it possible to get the protein that you need. Proteins can also be obtained from soybeans, nut butters, and tofu.

Variations on Meals—Ethnic Considerations

The U.S.A. is a melting pot of different cultures and the foods that most pregnant women eat are equally diverse. Many foods that you regularly eat may not be listed in the blocks. The way things are cooked or the spices used in cooking them will vary among cultures. For example, whether rice is Spanish, Persian, Indian, or Asian, it is still rice. The difference will be in what was added and how the rice was prepared. Spices add no calories, but oil, butter, lard, and margarine do. In order to include your favorite dishes in the food blocks, you will have to separate the individual components of the dish and place each in the appropriate groups. Then decide if they fit into the A, B, or C block of that group.

For example, a taco:

- Soft corn tortilla (A-block starch) vs. fried taco shell (C-block starch)

- White meat chicken (A-block meat) vs. dark meat (B-block meat)

- Black beans (A-block starch) vs. refried beans (C-block starch)

- Lettuce and tomatoes (A block)

Another example, Asian foods:

- Steamed brown rice (A-block starch) vs. fried rice (C-block starch)

- Steamed fish with sweet-and-sour sauce on the side (A-block meat) vs. whole fried fish (C-block meat)

- Steamed vegetables (free vegetable block) vs. stir-fried vegetables in peanut oil (count as both a vegetable and an A-block fat)

- Steamed vegetable dumplings (B-block starch and vegetable) vs. fried vegetable eggroll (C-block starch, A-block fat and vegetable)

■ The Milk Blocks ■

A MILK BLOCKS

Milk, nonfat . . . . .1 cup
Milk, 1 percent (low-fat) .1 cup
Buttermilk (low-fat) . . . . .1 cup
Evaporated milk, nonfat .½ cup
Dry milk, nonfat . . . . .⅓ cup (dry)
Yogurt, plain (nonfat) . . . . .1 cup
Soy milk, nonfat . . . . .1 cup

B MILK BLOCKS

Milk, reduced fat . . . . .1 cup
Milk, 2 percent . . . . .1 cup
Milk, chocolate, nonfat . . . . .1 cup
Evaporated milk, low-fat .½ cup
Dry milk, low-fat . . . . .⅓ cup (dry)
Yogurt, plain (low-fat) . . . . .1 cup
Yogurt, flavored . . . . .1 cup
Yogurt, fruited . . . . .1 cup
Soy milk, fortified low-fat . . . . .1 cup

C MILK BLOCKS

Milk, whole . . . . .1 cup
Milk, 4 percent . . . . .1 cup
Milk, chocolate, low-fat . . . . .1 cup
Evaporated milk, whole . . . . .½ cup
Yogurt, whole milk, ...1 cup

■ The Meat Blocks ■

A MEAT BLOCKS

Chicken/turkey, white meat (no skin) . . . . .1 oz
Fish and shellfish . . . . .1 oz
Tuna, canned (water-packed) .¼ cup
Salmon, canned (water-packed) . . . . .¼ cup
Cottage cheese, low-fat or nonfat . . . . .¼ cup
Egg whites . . . . .2 to 3
Egg substitute . . . . .¼ cup
Beans, peas, lentils . . . . .1 cup
Parmesan cheese, grated . . . . .2 T.
Cheese (3 or less grams of fat) . . . . .1 oz
Lamb, chop or leg . . . . .1 oz
Beef, lean (round, sirloin, tenderloin) . . . . .1 oz
Beef (flank, T-bone, ground round) . . . . .1 oz
Pork (ham or tenderloin) . . . . .1 oz
Canadian bacon . . . . .1 oz
Ricotta cheese, non or low-fat . . . . .¼ cup
Tofu (light) . . . . .½ cup
Soybeans . . . . .⅔ cup shelled

B MEAT BLOCKS

Chicken/turkey, dark meat
 (no skin) . . . . .1 oz
Beef (ground, meat loaf, short ribs,
 prime rib (no visible fat), lean
 brisket) .1 oz
Pork (chop or cutlets, not breaded) 1 oz
Veal cutlet (not breaded) . . . . .1 oz
Hot dogs (low-fat) 1
Meatballs .1 oz
Peanut butter (low-fat) . . . . .2 T.
Ricotta cheese . . . . .¼ cup
Mozzarella, string cheese . . . . . . .1 oz
Tofu . . . . .¼ cup
Egg 1

C MEAT BLOCKS

Fish, chicken, or pork (fried) . . . . .1 oz
Chicken, dark/white meat
 (skin on) . . . . .1 oz
Pork spare ribs . . . . .1 oz
Beef, luncheon meats (pastrami,
 salami, corned beef) . . . . .1 oz
Hot dogs (all regular) 1
Pork (pork sausage or spare ribs) . .1 oz
Veal cutlet (breaded) . . . . .1 oz
Peanut butter, almond butter . . . . .2 T.
Cheese, all regular (American,
 Cheddar, Swiss, Jack,
 Muenster) . . . . .1 oz

■ The Fruit Blocks ■

A FRUIT BLOCKS

1 small- to medium-size:	½ Fruit	1 cup	1 large
Apple	Banana	Berries	Kiwi
Peach	Papaya	Watermelon	Tangerine
Orange	Mango	Cantaloupe	Plum (or 2 small)
Pear	Grapefruit	Cherries	
	Grapes (½ cup)	Pineapple	

B FRUIT BLOCKS

Apricots . . . . .4 dried
Dates 3
Figs 2
Canned fruits
 (drained/juice-packed) . . . . . .½ cup
Raisins . . . . .2 T.
Cranberries (dry) . . . . .2 T.

C FRUIT BLOCKS

Apple juice . . . . .½ cup
Orange juice . . . . .½ cup
Grapefruit juice . . . . .½ cup
Pineapple juice . . . . .½ cup
Smoothie (all fruit) . . . . .½ cup
Cranberry juice . . . . .⅓ cup
Grape juice . . . . .⅓ cup
Prune juice . . . . .⅓ cup

■ The Vegetable Block ■

Enjoy any of these to your hearts content when eating them raw,
steamed, grilled, or broiled without added fat!

A VEGETABLE BLOCK

Artichoke	Celery	Onions	Spinach
Asparagus	Cucumber	Leeks	Water chestnuts
Carrots	Tomato	Mushrooms	Turnips
Broccoli	Eggplant	Bean sprouts	Vegetable juices (½ cup)
String beans	Peppers	Peapods	
Cabbage	Lettuce and salad greens	Squash (zucchini, crookneck)	

■ The Starch Blocks ■

A STARCH BLOCKS

Cereals (hot and cold):

All-Bran	½ cup
All-Bran Buds	⅓ cup
Shredded wheat and bran cereal	½ cup
Cheerios	¾ cup
Bran flakes	½ cup
Barbara's Puffins	¾ cup
Grape-Nuts	¼ cup
Puffed cereals	1½ cup
Wheat germ	3 T.
Hot oatmeal, oatbran, Cream of Wheat/Rice, grits	½ cup

Pasta/Rice/Potatoes/Beans/Vegetables:

Pasta (whole wheat or regular)	½ cup
Rice (steamed brown or white)	⅓ cup
Beans (black, kidney, white, pinto, lentils, black-eyed peas)	½ cup
Buckwheat groats	½ cup
Peas	½ cup
Corn	½ cup or 1 medium ear
Potato, baked	½ of a medium
Potato, mashed	½ cup
Squash (butternut and acorn)	1 cup
Yam	½ cup
Barley	½ cup

Breads and Crackers:

Bagel, mini	1 each
Bagel	½ small
Bread, wheat, white, rye, sourdough	1 slice (1 oz)
English muffin, whole wheat/white	½
Pita bread, whole-wheat or white	½
Bun, hamburger or hot dog	½
Crackers, low-fat or fat-free	3–6
Rice or corn cakes	2
Saltine crackers	6
Matzoh	¾ sheet or ¾ oz
Melba toast	5 rectangles, 5–10 rounds
Tortilla, large flour	½
Dinner roll	1 oz
Raisin bread	1 slice

A STARCH BLOCK SNACKS

Popcorn, air-popped or light microwave	3 cups
Graham cracker squares (regular, cinnamon or chocolate flavor)	3 squares
Pretzel	¾ oz or 1 medium

B STARCH BLOCK

Breakfast foods

Granola (lowfat)	¼ cup
Pancakes	2
Waffle, toaster whole wheat	1

Snacks

Cracker with fat	4–6
Angel food cake	1 oz.
Cookies, fat-free (equals 80–100 calories)	1–2
Fat-free granola bar (equals 80–100 calories)	1
Vanilla wafers	4
Teddy Grahams	13

C STARCH BLOCKS

Fried taco shell	1
Refried beans	½ cup
Fried rice	⅓ cup
Biscuit	1 each
Corn bread	2 oz.
French fries	10
Baby muffin	1 oz.
Stuffing	¼ cup

■ The Fat Blocks ■

A FAT BLOCKS

Avocado . . . . .⅛
Oil (canola and olive) . . . . .1 t.
Nuts (almonds, cashews, mixed) 6
Peanuts 10
Walnuts, pecans . . . . .4 halves
Seeds (pumpkin, sunflower, sesame) . . . . .1 T.

B FAT BLOCKS

Butter, light . . . . .1 T.
Margarine, low-fat . . . . .1 T.
Salad dressing, low-fat . . . . .2 T.
Sour cream, low-fat . . . . .3 T.
Cream cheese, low-fat . . . . .2 T.
Mayonnaise, low-fat . . . . .1 T.
Miracle Whip (light) . . . . .1 T.

C FAT BLOCKS

Bacon . . . . .1 slice
Butter . . . . .1 t.
Margarine . . . . .1 t.
Salad dressing (regular) . . . . .1 T.
Shortening or lard . . . . .1 t.
Sour cream (regular) . . . . .2 T.
Cream cheese (regular) . . . . .1 T.
Mayonnaise (regular) . . . . .1 t.
Miracle Whip . . . . .2 t.

Individualized Food Plans

Most pregnant women ask us for ideas about what to eat. Some would like us to supply the food, but that's impossible. Sample menu ideas are the next best thing. People always want new ideas about meals. One easy way to accomplish this is to rework our clients' current menus by replacing some foods with healthier alternatives.

Your doctor or dietitian will determine the amount of calories you need per day based on several factors. These include your prepregnant weight, current weight, fluctuations, and weight gain during previous pregnancies.

As a basic guide, we have included five 2,200-calorie menu plans that you can use in planning your meals. If you are following the 2,200-calorie meal plans, we suggest that you eat foods from each block as indicated at each meal. Feel free to move foods around to better suit your daily routine, and to substitute foods that you like better within each block. *In other words, don't leave out any of the blocks or you will not be getting enough nourishment for your developing baby.*

Remember, some women need more than 2,200 calories and others need less. The calories you will need as your pregnancy progresses will be determined by your actual weight gain over time. Your doctor or dietitian can help evaluate this.

As a reminder, your calcium requirement is met with milk from the milk block or cheese from the meat block. If you use neither, you can substitute calcium-fortified soy milk and soy cheese. If you don't use either soy or dairy products, then add an additional ounce of meat and take calcium pills.

Vegetarians can easily substitute many foods for their meat and milk blocks. These include tofu, soybeans, and other beans for protein. Calcium-fortified soy milk and soy milk products also can help you meet your calcium requirement.

Menu 1—2,200 Calories

Breakfast

2 STARCHES:	1 whole-wheat English muffin
2 MEATS:	2 eggs or 4 egg whites
VEGETABLES:	mushrooms, tomatoes, onions (for omelet or on side)
1 FRUIT:	1 orange cut into wedges
1 MILK:	8 oz nonfat or 1 percent milk
2 FATS:	2 T. BUTTER, MARGARINE, OR OIL

Midmorning Snack

1 STARCH:	2 rice cakes (any variety)
1 FRUIT:	1 peach

Lunch

2 STARCHES:	2 SLICES WHOLE-WHEAT BREAD OR WHOLE PITA
3 MEATS:	3 oz grilled chicken breast
VEGETABLES:	tomatoes, lettuce
1 FRUIT:	1 pear
2 FATS:	2 t. reg mayo, 2 T. light mayo, or 1/4 avocado

Midafternoon Snack (the sticks)

1 STARCH:	3/4 oz pretzel sticks
1 MEAT:	1 oz string cheese
VEGETABLE:	any "sticks" (carrot, jicama, cucumber, zucchini)

Dinner

2 STARCHES:	2/3 cup brown rice (steamed in chicken or vegetable broth)
4 MEATS:	4 oz lean, broiled steak (like small filet)
VEGETABLES:	steamed broccoli or cauliflower
1 FRUIT:	baked apple or 1/2 cup natural applesauce
2 FATS:	2 t. olive oil or butter (use on vegetables or salad)

Evening Snack

1 STARCH:	3 graham-cracker squares
1/2 MEAT:	1 T. peanut or almond butter
1 MILK:	8 oz nonfat or 1 percent milk

Menu 2—2,200 Calories

Breakfast

2 STARCHES:	1/4 cup Grape-Nuts cereal + 1/4 cup low-fat granola
2 MEATS:	1/2 cup cottage cheese
1 FRUIT:	1 cup mixed berries (fresh or frozen)
1 MILK:	8 oz nonfat or low-fat plain yogurt
1 FAT:	6 chopped roasted almonds

Midmorning Snack

1 STARCH:	1 mini raisin bagel
1/2 MEAT:	1 T. peanut, almond, or soy butter

Lunch

2 STARCHES:	2 slices whole-wheat bread or whole pita
3 MEATS:	3 oz sliced turkey breast
VEGETABLES:	tomatoes, lettuce
1 FRUIT:	2 small tangerines
2 FATS:	2 t. regular mayo, 1 T. light mayo, or 1/4 avocado
1 MILK:	8 oz nonfat or 1 percent milk

Midafternoon Snack

1 STARCH:	8 animal crackers
1 MILK:	8 oz nonfat or 1 percent milk

Dinner (burger night)

3 STARCHES:	1 whole-wheat bun and "fake fries" from 1/2 medium potato
4 MEATS:	4 oz lean ground beef, turkey, chicken, fish, or vegetable patty
VEGETABLES:	lettuce, tomato, onion
1 FRUIT:	1 1/4 cup watermelon cubes
2 FATS:	2 t. regular mayo, 2 T. light mayo, or 1/4 avocado

Evening Snack: (A real treat)

1 STARCH:	3 graham crackers, crumbled
1 FRUIT:	1/2 banana
1 MILK:	1/2 cup nonfat or low-fat frozen yogurt

Menu 3—2,200 Calories

Breakfast (bagel breakfast)

2 STARCHES:	2 mini raisin bagels or 1 "toaster" bagel (2–3 oz smaller bagel)
2 MEATS:	½ cup cottage cheese topped with cinnamon
1 FRUIT:	1 cup cantaloupe
1 MILK:	8 oz nonfat or 1 percent milk

Midmorning Snack (quesadilla snack)

1 STARCH:	1 corn tortilla
1 MEAT:	1 oz light cheese, melted
VEGETABLE:	chopped tomato or salsa

Lunch

2 STARCHES:	2 slices whole-wheat bread or whole pita
3 MEATS:	¾ cup canned, water-packed tuna or salmon
VEGETABLES:	tomatoes, lettuce
1 FRUIT:	17 small grapes or 1 dozen larger grapes
2 FATS:	2 t. regular mayo, 1 T. light mayo, or ¼ avocado
1 MILK:	8 oz nonfat or 1 percent milk

Midafternoon Snack

1 STARCH:	low-fat wheat crackers that equal 80–100 calories per serving
1 MEAT:	1 oz low-fat, pasteurized soft-cheese cubes (ex. Laughing Cow)

Dinner (Asian delight)

2 STARCHES:	1 cup noodles or ⅔ cup rice (try brown rice)
4 MEATS:	4 oz lean beef or chicken strips, stir-fried (see fat)
VEGETABLES:	assorted peppers, onion, bean sprouts, and carrots
1 FRUIT:	½ cup canned mandarin oranges or 2 small tangerines
2 FATS:	2 t. peanut or sesame oil for stir frying

Evening Snack

2 FATS:	12 almonds or cashews
1 FRUIT:	2 T. or small box raisins

Menu 4—2,200 Calories

Breakfast (high-fiber)

2 STARCHES:	1/2 cup All-Bran or All-Bran Buds + 1/2 cup shredded-wheat-and-bran cereal
1 FRUIT:	1 cup mixed berries (fresh or frozen)
1 MILK:	8 oz nonfat or 1 percent milk
1 FAT:	6 chopped roasted almonds

Midmorning Snack

1 STARCH:	whole-wheat pretzel
1 MEAT:	1 hard-boiled egg
VEGETABLES:	grape or cherry tomatoes

Lunch (pizza day)

2 STARCHES:	1 whole-wheat English muffin or mini pizza shell (Boboli)
3 MEATS:	3 oz shredded mozzarella (low-fat)
VEGETABLES:	tomatoes, mushrooms, and 1/4 cup marinara sauce
1 FRUIT:	1/2 cup fresh or canned pineapple (can be added to pizza)
1 MILK:	8 oz nonfat or 1 percent milk

Midafternoon Snack

1 STARCH:	8 animal crackers
1/2 MILK	1/2 cup fat-free pudding or homemade pudding with non-fat milk

Dinner (Mexican night)

3 STARCHES:	1 cup black bean soup + 1 toasted corn tortilla
4 MEATS:	3 oz lean beef, turkey, chicken + 1 oz low-fat cheese, shredded
1 FAT:	1 T. dressing with tossed green salad
VEGETABLES:	diced onions, peppers, tomato (for tortilla) + salsa
1 FRUIT:	1/2 papaya
2 FATS:	2 t. oil, 1/4 avocado, or 6 T. light sour cream

Evening Snack: (smoothie)

FREE:	ice cubes to blend the fruit and yogurt
1 FRUIT:	1/2 banana
1/2 MILK	4 oz vanilla yogurt

Menu 5—2,200 Calories

Breakfast (it's hot!)

2 STARCHES:	1 cup hot oatmeal or Cream of Wheat (measure 1 cup after cooking)
1 FRUIT:	2 T. raisins
1 MILK:	8 oz nonfat or 1 percent milk
1 FAT:	6 chopped roasted almonds or 1 t. butter or margarine

Midmorning Snack

1 FRUIT:	sliced fresh apple
½ MEAT:	1 T. peanut, almond, or soy butter
1 STARCH:	28 Goldfish pretzel crackers

Lunch

2 STARCHES:	1 medium baked potato or yam
3 MEATS:	¾ cup cottage cheese or vegetarian chili
VEGETABLES:	broccoli, green onions, and tomato salsa
1 FRUIT:	1 cup honeydew
2 FATS:	2 t. butter or margarine or 6 T. light sour cream
1 MILK:	8 oz nonfat or 1 percent milk or 1 oz shredded light cheese (for potato)

Midafternoon Snack

1 STARCH:	3 cups popcorn (air-popped or light microwave)

Dinner (Italian night)

2 STARCHES:	1 cup pasta
4 MEATS:	4 oz poached salmon or other allowed fish
VEGETABLES:	fresh salad + green beans
1 FRUIT:	⅓ cantaloupe
2 FATS:	2 t. olive oil (for pasta or to sauté garlic) or 4 T. light dressing
FREE:	nonfat salad dressing, lemon juice, or balsamic vinegar
1 MILK:	8 oz nonfat or 1 percent milk

Evening Snack

1 STARCH:	6–8 mini rice cakes
1 MEAT:	1 oz low-fat cheese
1 FRUIT:	frozen-fruit-juice bar (about 100 calories)

If you follow this guide and find that you need to change the calories, refer to the notes below. One last comment: if you have food allergies to any items in the sample menus, refer to the food blocks for alternate choices.

How to Adjust the Calorie Level of Your Meal Plan

We call these our simple math menus because if you are gaining too fast or not gaining enough, you can add or subtract 200 calories in either direction by using the food blocks below. Eliminate or add foods in the following manner:

1 Starch (80 calories)

1 Meat (55–100 calories)

1 Fat (45 calories)

Take off or add the above to any meal during the day. If you need to add additional calories, you can add a snack or simply have more food at one meal.

A second way to add calories is by drinking an additional glass of milk once or twice a day (approximately 90 to 120 calories). This will add protein, carbohydrates, calcium, and a little fat (1 percent milk) without causing you to eat more solid food.

The third option is to keep the number of servings per block stable but be careful how you choose foods from the food blocks. If you need to reduce your intake, choose primarily A-block foods. If you need to increase your calories, choose foods from the B and C blocks.

Although we normally discourage beverages with calories,

if you are not feeling well and are not gaining enough weight, this would be the time to add juices, milk shakes, and smoothies.

Foods to Use with Caution

It's not our intention to scare you but to inform you about the dangers of eating certain types of food. Being a little cautious for nine months is well worth it in the end. We have listed these foods based on the food blocks that you learned about earlier in this chapter. Be sure to check with your doctor for the final word regarding these foods.

FOODS TO AVOID IN EACH BLOCK

The milk/yogurt blocks

- Nonpasteurized or raw milk. *(Rationale: these products can be contaminated with toxic* E. coli *bacteria.)*

- Soft cheeses, including feta, Brie, Camembert, bleu cheese, and Mexican-style cheeses. *(Rationale: eating these cheeses may cause listeriosis, which is a bacterial infection caused by* Listeria monocytogenes.)

The meat blocks

- Processed meats (including hot dogs and cold cuts). Because these foods are usually high in salt, fat, and contain nitrites, we do not recommend that you select from this group. However, if you occasionally choose these processed meats, do not eat them cold; they must be thoroughly heated. *(Rationale: there is a minor concern that eating these foods can cause listeriosis.)*

■ Raw or undercooked beef, especially ground beef. *(Rationale: there is a concern that these foods can be contaminated with toxic* E. coli *bacteria.)*

■ Something's fishy! When we were pregnant, there was nothing fishy about eating fish! In fact, after the nausea was over, we had tuna sandwiches on a regular basis in our lunch bags. Now things are different, and you should include fish in your diet but limit, or completely avoid, certain fish.

▪ Raw fish and seafood (sushi) should be eliminated. *(Rationale: these fish can be contaminated with methyl mercury, PBCs (lead), i.e., bacterial and viral contamination.)*

▪ According to the American Dietetic Association's Diet Manual,[1] fatty fish such as swordfish, shark, and fresh and frozen tuna should be limited to one time per month. According to the FDA's food safety Website, in addition to the fish above, king mackerel and tilefish should also be avoided. This site also suggested limiting all other fish to a total of 12 ounces or less per week. *(Rationale: these fish can be contaminated with methyl mercury and PBCs.)*

▪ Trout and other large, older lake fish should be limited to once per month. *(Rationale: these fish can be contaminated with methyl mercury and PBCs.)*

▪ Canned tuna can also be contaminated with methyl mercury, and some sources say you should limit your intake of tuna to once per week; others say once per month.[2] To be safe, we recommend that you check with your doctor and eat a variety of safe fish in moderation.

▪ Local fish. If you have an occasion to eat fish caught locally, be sure to check out its safety on the Web site or by calling phone number listed below:

1(888)SAFEFOOD
Food and Drug Administration Web site:
www.cfsan.fda.gov

■ Raw or undercooked poultry. *(Rationale: these foods can be contaminated with salmonella bacteria.)*

■ Raw or soft-cooked eggs. *(Rationale: these foods can be contaminated with salmonella bacteria.)*

The fruit blocks

■ Unwashed fruits and vegetables. Before you cut into that great looking melon, remember that you must wash it. It's not a good idea to take your knife and push the bacteria from the outside into the "meat" of the juicy, ripe melon. Using a good fruit/vegetable brush, scrub the surface of your melon under cold, running water. Washing it thoroughly should get off any surface dirt and make it safe to eat. There are also other vegetable "washes" that you can buy at the market. Check them out! *(Rationale: eating these foods [before they are washed] could cause you to become infected with salmonella bacteria. Melons grow in soil that is often fertilized with manure.)*

■ Unpasteurized juices such as apple cider. *(Rationale: these foods can be contaminated with toxic* E. coli *bacteria.)*

Chapter Ten

Managing Your Weight While You Wait!

Now that you are familiar with the food building blocks, you can monitor your diet and your weight gain by learning about some practical tools. These tools will help you implement the food recommendations of the previous chapter without much difficulty. We recommend that everyone use the weight-gain graph, food diary, and food checklist described in this chapter.

Monitoring Your Weight Gain: Your Weight-Gain Graph

One of the most important things to ask your doctor is to set the weight-gain-goal range for your pregnancy. Figure 1 shows a simple chart that records your prepregnancy weight, number of weeks pregnant, and your actual weight gain. After writing down these numbers, mark off your appropriate weight-range goal on the right side of the graph (see figure 2). You can record the actual weight gain either on your own or in conjunction with your doctor appointments. When you see your doctor or nurse practitioner, bring along the graph so that your weight can be recorded. This graph will allow both you and your doctor to measure your progress. We have also included samples of 3 typical weight gain graphs so that you can see how weight gain varies from person to person.

Graph 1: This graph illustrates the weight-gain pattern of a woman who suffered from severe morning sickness and lost about 7 pounds in the first trimester. Once she was feeling better, her weight quickly increased and then leveled off in the last trimester, with a total weight gain of 34 pounds. She regained the 7 pounds she lost, plus 27 more.

Graph 2: This graph illustrates the weight gain of a woman who started her pregnancy at a weight of 180 pounds. She suffered some nausea and found that the best solution was to keep eating small meals all day long until the nausea subsided. She was able to keep her weight gain under control for the remainder of the pregnancy. She gained 35 pounds total.

Graph 3: This graph represents the weight gain of a five-foot four-inch woman whose weight prior to each of her two pregnancies was 200 pounds. She had a difficult time dieting prior to both the first and second pregnancies, but seemed to be in great control during each of the pregnancies. She said it was because she was "not that hungry." To us, it appeared that she was making a conscientious effort to watch what she was eating. Her weight-gain graph was exactly what we wanted it to look like, and it was almost identical in both pregnancies. She continues to work on keeping her weight under control as a mom of two.

Prenatal Weight Chart

Figure 1

Prepregnant weight: _____

Date	Weeks Gestation	Weight	Total Weight Gain

Pregnancy Weight-Gain Graph

Figure 2

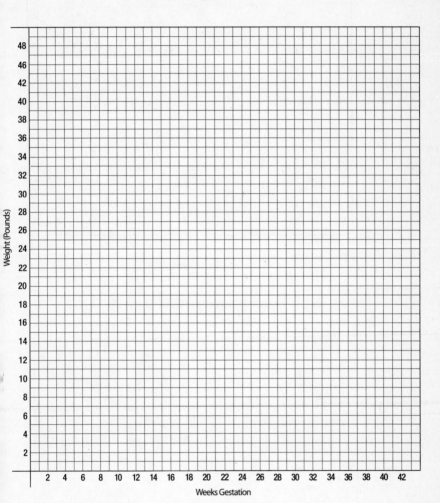

Pregnancy Weight Gain Graph 1

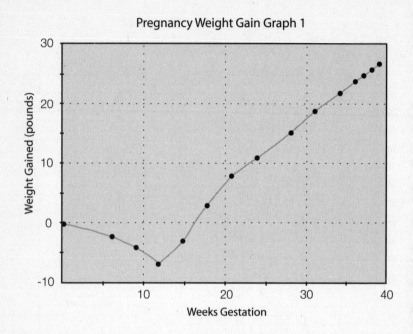

Pregnancy Weight Gain Graph 2

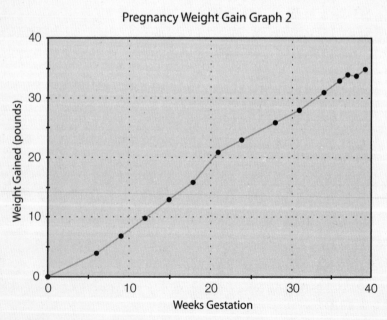

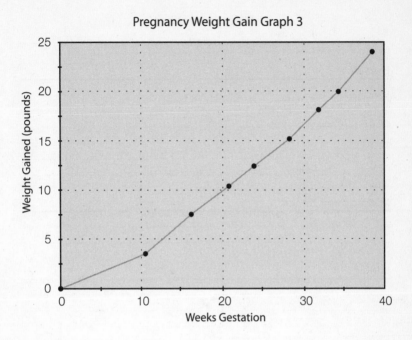

Daily Food Diary

Now that you are familiar with the weight-gain graph, the next tool will help you keep track of what you are eating. One of the best ways to be aware of your eating patterns is to write down everything that you eat and drink. We know this is very tedious and bothersome, but in the end, awareness of your food choices is worth every bit of the time it takes. One suggestion is to try to write down the foods you are planning to eat *before* you eat them. This helps you make deliberate choices rather than impulsive ones.

You can make multiple photocopies of the Daily Food Diary page to record your foods.

Daily Food Diary

Figure 3

Breakfast:

_____
_____
_____
_____
_____
_____

Midmorning Snack:

_____
_____

Lunch:

_____
_____
_____
_____

Midafternoon Snack:

_____
_____

Dinner:

_____
_____
_____
_____
_____

Evening Snack:

_____
_____

Daily Food Diary: Sample

Figure 3

Breakfast:

4 oz orange juice

2 scrambled eggs

1 slice toast with butter and jelly

Decaf coffee/cream/sugar

Midmorning Snack:

1 apple

Lunch:

Tuna sandwich on wheat bread

Orange

Pretzels

Diet Coke

Midafternoon Snack:

Muffin and decaf

Dinner:

Green salad with Italian dressing

4 oz chicken breast

Baked potato, low fat sour cream

Asparagus

Sourdough bread with butter

Evening Snack:

Fruit ice pop

Accounting for Your Food: Daily Food-and-Fluid Checkoff Sheet

The final tool to monitor your nutritional status is the food-and-fluid checkoff sheet. You will transfer the information from your diary onto this sheet. Think of your daily food intake like a bank account. Each day you will have an allowance of foods from your food account. In order to not overeat in one food block, you can use this tool to gauge your nutritional intake. Some people will need more food and some will need less, and that is why we give you a range within each block. The symbols that correspond to each block will be based on a level of 2,200 to 2,400 calories per day. When you have used up the allowances in your food account, you can feel confident that you have eaten a well-balanced diet. When looking at the vegetable group, note that you can spend more because these foods are low in calories and high in fiber and nutrients. If you find that the food from your diary is either more or less than your allowance for the day, you will need to adjust up or down depending on your weight gain. (See the sample checkoff sheet.)

Shopping Tools

By using the extensive food blocks described in chapter 9, you can develop shopping lists to buy foods in your plan. The most important piece of advice about shopping is to plan your meals in advance. One useful way to do this is to sit down with your family and have everyone give suggestions about what they would like to eat over the next week. Once you write down their choices, you will avoid impulse buying followed by impulse eating. Remember: don't buy anything that you shouldn't eat even if it's on sale. This includes food that you

Weekly Food Check Off Sheet
Figure 4

SUNDAY
Starches (9–11) — — — — — — — — — — —
Meat (9–11) — — — — — — — — — — —
Fruit (3–4) — — — —
Milk (2–4) — — — —
Fat (6–7) — — — — — — —

MONDAY
Starches (9–11) — — — — — — — — — —
Meat (9–11) — — — — — — — — —
Fruit (3–4) — — — —
Milk (2–4) — — — —
Fat (6–7) — — — — — — —

TUESDAY
Starches (9–11) — — — — — — — — — —
Meat (9–11) — — — — — — — — — —
Fruit (3–4) — — — —
Milk (2–4) — — — —
Fat (6–7) — — — — — — —

WEDNESDAY
Starches (9–11) — — — — — — — — —
Meat (9–11) — — — — — — — — —
Fruit (3–4) — — — —
Milk (2–4) — — — —
Fat (6–7) — — — — —

THURSDAY
Starches (9–11) — — — — — — — — —
Meat (9–11) — — — — — — — — —
Fruit (3–4) — — — —
Milk (2–4) — — — —
Fat (6–7) — — — — — — —

FRIDAY
Starches (9–11) — — — — — — — — —
Meat (9–11) — — — — — — — — —
Fruit (3–4) — — — —
Milk (2–4) — — — —
Fat (6–7) — — — — — — —

SATURDAY
Starches (9–11) — — — — — — — — — —
Meat (9–11) — — — — — — — — — —
Fruit (3–4) — — — —
Milk (2–4) — — — —
Fat (6–7) — — — — — — —

Sample Food Check Off Sheet

Breakfast
4 oz Orange Juice
2 scrambled eggs
I slice toast with butter and jelly
Decaf Coffee/cream/sugar

Midmorning Snack
I apple

Lunch
Tuna sandwich on wheat bread
Orange
Pretzels
Diet Coke

Midafternoon Snack:
Muffin & Decaf

Dinner
Green salad with Italian dressing
4 oz. chicken breast
Baked potato, low-fat sour cream
Asparagus
Sourdough bread with butter

Evening Snack
Fruit ice pop

Starches (9–11)	X	X	X	X	X	X	X	X	X	X	X
Meat (9–11)	X	X	X	X	X	X	X	X	X		
Fruit (3–4)	X	X	X	X							
Milk (2–4)	none										
Fat (6–7)	X	X	X	X	X	X	X				

This daily checkoff sheet was based on the sample food diary in figure 3. An analysis of this sheet illustrates that this client had the appropriate amount of fruit, meat and fat. Unfortunately, she went over her allotment of starches and did not have any milk. We asked her about her calcium intake, since it was not represented in her food diary. She explained that she was taking four Tums-ex per day, (1200 milligrams of calcium). This was an acceptable amount of calcium, but she agreed to eat some plain yogurt (which contains 300 mg of calcium and 8 grams of protein) with some fresh fruit and skip one of the Tums-ex. Lastly, we recommended that she skip the muffin (which represented four starches and two fats), and choose graham crackers or rice cakes instead. As an alternative, we suggested that she make her own, smaller-size, low-fat muffins.

think your family would like but you shouldn't have. If it's necessary to buy desserts, chips, or ice cream, buy these items in single-portion servings and store them in a space that is reserved just for them. Thus, in the event that you, too, decide to indulge, you will not have to make a choice about your portion size.

Kitchen Tools

We suggest that you keep the following tools handy on your counter. If they're visible, there is a good chance that you will use them.

- Measuring spoons
- Measuring cups
- Food scale

Chapter Eleven

Plus-Size Workout

Exercise in Pregnancy

There are two kinds of people in the world, the jocks and the couch potatoes. A jock adores exercise. It's her favorite recreational activity. Her day is not complete without a run or a swim, and she wouldn't dream of packing for a business trip or a vacation without including a pair of running shorts and sneakers. If a jock can't exercise for a few days, she becomes positively crabby. Given a free weekend, she'll always opt for a hike or a bike ride (rather than a good movie, or shopping).

Then there is the couch potato. No doubt she has read, and believes, that exercise helps produce cardiovascular fitness. She understands about the endorphin rush that's supposed to make you feel so energized. She just hasn't been able to find a form of exercise she truly loves enough to want to do daily. It's not that she doesn't try. Over the years she has probably ran, hiked, backpacked, swam, joined a gym, done aerobics, pumped iron, gone cross country skiing, bicycled, and used a treadmill. None of it comes close to the pleasure she experiences curled up with a really good book.

One thing people often don't understand is that it's a lot harder to exercise when you are overweight. Take a brisk walk around the block. Then do it again carrying a 40-pound backpack. That's what it feels like to exercise when you are overweight. You're off on a hike with your best buddies. They're moving along at a brisk pace, and you're huffing and puffing to keep up. You're out of breath, your heart is going a mile a minute, and you're sweating like a pig. This is not fun.

So why should you even consider exercising while you are pregnant? The answer is that labor is a huge athletic event. You wouldn't dream of running a marathon without training for it. Pushing a baby out requires cardiovascular fitness and endurance. It is the hardest physical work you will ever do in your life, and you want to be as ready for it as you can be. If you end up having a cesarean section, you don't want it to be because you were too exhausted to push. Modern technology can help you have a painless labor and can even take most of the pain away when you are pushing. Unfortunately, modern medicine has yet to figure out a way to push for you. It's the one part of childbirth that is 100 percent your job. If you are already reasonably fit and exercise regularly, your goal should be to maintain your current level of cardiovascular fitness. If you never exercise and consider yourself horribly out of shape, your goal should be to make some modest improvement in your endurance.

Do's and Don'ts of Exercising While Pregnant

- Do everything in moderation.

- If you've never run a marathon, don't start training for it now.

- Start slowly and build up gradually. Fifteen minutes a day is plenty if you've never exercised before. We know all those pregnancy exercise videotapes go on for an hour, but you don't have to do the whole thing at once.

- Check your pulse rate periodically. The American College of Obstetrics and Gynecology originally recommended a maximum heart rate of 140 beats per minute for exercising pregnant women. Although they subsequently eliminated the number, deciding it was too restrictive for women who were trained athletes, most overweight women aren't, and 140 beats per minute is a safe guideline.

- Don't exercise during the hottest part of the day, and if you feel yourself getting significantly overheated, tired, dizzy, or short of breath—just stop.

- Don't do sit-ups after the first trimester.

- Don't do any exercise that will strain your back or risk injury to your joints. Those parts of your body are particularly vulnerable when you are pregnant. Ordinarily your abdominal muscles help you to stand straight, but during pregnancy your abdominal muscles relax to allow your uterus to expand, and your back muscles work overtime. In addition, during the third trimester, the cartilage in your joints softens to allow your pelvis to spread. This makes your joints easier to damage. Be gentle to your body.

- High impact exercise should be avoided during the second and third trimester. Skip the snowboarding and the parachute jumps.

- Keep a water bottle handy and stay well hydrated.

- Don't exercise on your back after sixteen weeks gestation. The weight of the uterus will put pressure on your vena cava and decrease blood flow.

- Above all use common sense and stop if anything hurts.

What Kind of Exercise Is Best for Pregnant Women?

The best exercise for a pregnant woman is something she actually enjoys or at least doesn't hate. If you are an overscheduled working woman, it needs to be something you can easily make time for.

Swimming is great exercise if you are pregnant. The water helps support your weight and you don't get hot and sweaty. You do, of course, need easy access to a pool, and dealing with your hair afterward can be time-consuming.

Walking is easy and works for everyone. A treadmill in front of the TV for twenty minutes a day is boring, but it gets the job done. A quick walk through the neighborhood is even better. It's best if you can find a walking partner. We recommend dogs. They are loyal, loving, always available, and willing to walk at your pace. Of course they do insist on sniffing at every lamppost and periodically they urinate on the neighbors' grass, but they never outrun you and they never make snide comments about how out of shape you are.

Jogging, with appropriate modifications of distance and pace, can usually be done comfortably through the second trimester. After that, having a large pregnant belly bouncing up and down is pretty uncomfortable and will throw your balance off. If you are already a runner, by all means continue, but take it easy. If you've never run before, stick to a brisk walk instead.

Low-impact aerobics are excellent pregnancy exercises. Try one of the many pregnancy exercise videos such as the one produced by Kathy Smith.[1] The advantage to a video is that you can do whatever portion you like best for as long as you like. For those folks who are in better shape and can work out for an hour, there are lots of pregnancy exercise classes offered by gyms, YWCAs, and even hospitals.

Yoga helps build strength and flexibility. There are many different schools of yoga, and the positions taught vary from very easy to impossibly difficult even in the nonpregnant state. Keep in mind our warnings about back and joint injury. If you wish to do yoga during pregnancy, you are best off taking a class with a very experienced teacher designed specifically for pregnant women. Use common sense and stop immediately if anything you are doing begins to hurt.

Bicycling is a good way to build cardiovascular endurance and is safe during pregnancy whether you use a stationary bike or actually get outdoors. As you reach your third trimester, balance may become a problem on a nonstationary bike, and you may wish to switch to another form of exercise.

Weight training can be done during early pregnancy with a few caveats. You are best off working out with very light weights and more repetitions. Don't try to bench-press 200 pounds. You'd hate to slip and have the weights land on your stomach. Don't lift anything heavy that requires effort from your back muscles. That's also asking for trouble. As you get more pregnant, you might be better off switching to a different kind of exercise. Remember, your joints are weaker and more easily strained.

Special Concerns for the Extremely Overweight

Just being pregnant puts an extra strain on your heart and lungs. Sometimes you get so out of breath that it feels as if you've run a mile, even though you've been sitting down for the past hour. These are normal changes. However, for women who are extremely overweight, the added burden of pregnancy can push cardiac capacity to its upper limits, so that even normal daily activity is an effort.

Experts in exercise physiology recommend a range of target heart rates during exercise that are correlated to age. Kathy Smith, in her pregnancy exercise video, suggests the following heart rate range.[2]

Age	Heart Rate beats/min
20–25	120–138
26–30	114–136
31–35	108–132
36–40	108–126

The goal is to keep your heart rate at 60 to 70 percent of the maximum while you are working out. A good rule of thumb is that you should be able to carry on a conversation while you are exercising.

The problem with these particular numbers is that they are meant for women who are not excessively heavy. We define how hard a heart is working by the term "cardiac output." This is the volume of blood pumped each time the heart contracts multiplied by the number of contractions per minute. A heart muscle that is very fit will be able to pump a larger volume of blood with each contraction, and will therefore not need to pump as many times per minute to deliver the amount of oxygen needed by the body. In-shape athletes usually have very low heart rates. The amount of oxygen your body needs depends on your size, so that a heavy person needs a heart that contracts more efficiently or faster than a thin person. A 150-pound pregnant woman may have a baseline heart rate of 70. A 250-pound woman may have a baseline heart rate of 90. Her heart is already beating harder and faster just to supply all her extra tissues. For someone that heavy, these target rates are probably too high. Unfortunately, there are no specific guidelines that modify these numbers based on BMI. We recommend staying very much at the low end of the target.

Contraindications to Exercise in Pregnancy

According to the American College of Obstetrics and Gynecology (ACOG),[3] you should not exercise if you have any of the following:

- Pregnancy-induced hypertension

- Premature rupture of the membranes

- Preterm labor during the current or previous pregnancy

- A prematurely dilated cervix requiring a suture called a cerclage to keep it closed

- Any second- or third-trimester bleeding

- A baby with intrauterine growth retardation

Before embarking on any exercise program during pregnancy, be sure to discuss your plans and concerns with your doctor and get your doctor's approval. This is particularly important for women who are very obese. If you and your physician agree that some exercise is a good idea, pick something very easy, like walking or swimming, and start very slowly. Even if you are only moderately overweight, you should still clear your exercise regimen with your obstetrician.

Chapter Twelve

Medical Nutrition Therapy

When to See a Dietitian

Most women are able to carry a pregnancy without requiring intervention from a dietitian. However, there are instances when a doctor may recommend medical nutrition therapy to address some common nutritional concerns during pregnancy.

Nausea and Vomiting

The dietitian coauthors of this book have had lots of experience with nausea and vomiting. Between the two of us, we had five pregnancies with nausea and vomiting. One of our first bonding experiences was when Marlene walked into Netty's office as Netty was leaning over a trash can. Marlene had just returned from maternity leave only to find out that Netty was pregnant (again). When Marlene saw the look on Netty's face, she knew.

The secret was out. Marlene quickly ran to get some crackers, thinking of the "old cure," but it didn't help. What helps? What helps for one woman may not work for another. In fact, what works one day may not work the next day. Trial and error is the way to go. Remember, morning (or even noon and night sickness) is a temporary state. It usually lasts for not much longer than the first trimester or the first half of the pregnancy, but it often seems like a lifetime. If you feel that you cannot keep anything down, especially fluids, call your doctor immediately for assistance. Do not take any over-the-counter antinausea medication without your doctor's approval. As with most pregnancies, one day the morning sickness will be "magically" gone and you'll feel great. After it's over, be sure to get back to eating as healthfully as possible.

Here are some suggestions that we recommend. Not everything will work for you, but it's worth a try to help beat your nausea.

- Eat every three hours. It will keep your blood sugar at a good level. Quite often when the blood sugar drops, you get nauseated. Or is it the empty stomach?

- Try eating your food without drinking any beverage. After a short period of time, try *sipping* on liquids instead of drinking large quantities. This is particularly helpful when you are already feeling nauseous. Give bubbly water a try, too.

- Eat more when you are feeling better. If you feel better in the afternoon, make that the time you eat your bigger meal.

- If you crave sweet foods during this morning-sickness period, eat them. Try to choose fruit-juice bars, dried fruit, juice on ice, graham crackers, or animal crackers.

These choices are lower in calories than candy bars or regular cookies but achieve the same goals.

■ If you are craving salty foods, have soups, crackers, pretzels, and rice cakes that have some added salt.

■ Take your prenatal vitamin after lunch or dinner rather than in the morning. Usually, with food in your stomach, tolerating the vitamin is easier. If you still have difficulty with this supplement, it is best to ask your doctor about taking individual vitamins or minerals rather than a multivitamin supplement.

■ Make sure to have plenty of fluids. You might have to replace the fluids you are losing if you are vomiting or feeling dehydrated. Sipping fluids or fruit-juice pops in between meals will help keep you hydrated.

■ Though you are trying to keep your weight gain under control, during this time, eat what you can and worry about following the plans when you are feeling better.

■ Try to avoid strong odors, especially if you have to cook! This may be a good time to let your significant other do the cooking or get your family and friends to pitch in and help.

■ Try Sea-Bands.

■ If you feel somewhat relieved after vomiting, try eating small amounts of food.

■ Take the entire day to eat your food if you need to. Don't think in terms of meals.

■ If you're up to it, try looking through recipe books or magazines to see what looks appetizing. Once you find something, go for it!

■ If you can get out of bed, try eating your meals outdoors, such as in a park, where you'll get lots of fresh air.

Multiple Births

With multiple births, you have to gain more! This means you have to eat a little more. Check with your doctor early in the pregnancy to find out your weight-gain goal. Most of our patients gain somewhere between 7 to 10 extra pounds with twins. One important fact to remember is that you must take not only the weight of the other baby into consideration but also the placenta, amniotic fluid, and other tissues needed to support the pregnancy. In the plus pregnancy with extra babies, your doctor would probably recommend a weight gain of 25 to 35 pounds. What does this mean in food terms? According to the American Dietetic Association Diet Manual,[1] you should include an additional 150 calories per day over what you would need for a single pregnancy. What does that mean in terms of food? One extra piece of toast and one extra piece of string cheese or an extra glass of milk and three-quarters of a cup of cereal. It is as simple as adding an extra healthy snack. You will definitely be hungry when carrying a little extra becomes a lot extra. Keep in mind, the final say on weight gain with a multiple pregnancy needs to come from your doctor.

Bowels of Pregnancy

Even if you have a digestive system that works like a charm when you're not pregnant, be prepared for changes. A growing fetus pushes your bowels around and may cause some unforeseen nuisances. Constipation and diarrhea are two common complaints of many pregnant women.

CONSTIPATION

Many pregnant women complain about constipation. The two most important diet considerations to help alleviate constipation are the two *F*s: fluid and fiber! Having 25 to 35 grams of fiber per day should help considerably. Whatever you do, do not take laxatives or stool softeners unless prescribed by your doctor.

Since fiber loves fluid, try drinking eight to twelve glasses of calorie-free fluids per day. These can include water, decaffeinated iced tea, flavored carbonated water (without artificial sweeteners), or herbal teas. Flavor these drinks with a wedge of lemon, lime, or orange.

By including the high-fiber foods and fluid at the start of your pregnancy, you might be lucky enough to prevent hemorrhoids, which many women develop as their pregnancies progress. Please review the chart that follows to learn which foods are high in fiber and then incorporate them into your shopping lists and meal plan.

DIARRHEA

If you experience diarrhea during your pregnancy, treat it as you would if not pregnant. Drink plenty of fluids to replace those lost. Have broth, decaffeinated tea, diluted apple or cranberry juices, bubbly water, white rice, bananas, peeled apples or applesauce or the insides of a baked apple. Remember to check with your doctor if this lasts longer than a day.

EDEMA OR FLUID RETENTION

Many of our patients complain about fluid retention. They say they feel puffy, have trouble removing their rings, and want to know if they have to watch their salt intake. Most pregnant

Some Fiber Ideas!

	Fiber (grams)	Calories
Breakfast Cereals		
Post Shredded Wheat and Bran (½ c.)	4	100
Kellogg's All-Bran (½ c.)	10	80
Post 100% Bran (⅓ c.)	8	80
Barbara's Puffins (¾ c.)	5	90
Grape-Nuts cereal (¼ c.)	2.5	100
Quaker Toasted Oatmeal (½ c.)	2	95
Trader Joe's High Fiber Cereal (⅔ c.)	9	90
Quaker Instant Oatmeal, plain (1 packet)	3	80
Cheerios (1 c.)	2	100
Vegetables		
Broccoli (½ c. cooked)	3	25
Carrot (1 raw)	2	25
Spinach (½ c. cooked)	3	30
Tomato (½ c. cooked)	2	25
Sweet potato (1 small)	2	160
Fruits		
Raspberries (frozen) (1c.)	2	50
Orange (medium)	3	60
Nectarine (medium)	3	60

	Fiber (grams)	Calories
Fruits (continued)		
Pear (medium)	3	60
Prunes (5)	3	100
Beans and Peas (½ cup)		
Black beans	3.5	100
Lentils	4.0	115
Lima beans	3.9	115
Kidney beans	3.2	112
Garbanzo beans (chickpeas)	2.7	130
Soybeans (shelled)	4.0	100
Northern beans	3	100
Breads and Crackers		
Whole-wheat bread (1 slice)	2–3	80–90
Light whole-wheat bread (2 slices)	5–7	80–90
Reduced-fat Triscuit crackers (7)	4	120
Ak-mak Crackers (5)	3.5	116

women do not have to be concerned with this. Salt is needed during pregnancy and should not be restricted unless you are instructed to do so by your doctor. If you are weighing yourself at home and see a sudden rapid weight gain, call your doctor, who may want you to see you and check your blood pressure.

HYPERCHOLESTEROLEMIA

Sometimes women have preexisting high cholesterol. This is not something that you develop during the pregnancy. By following our guidelines and selecting the best choices within each food group, your diet will not be too high in fat or sugar. The recommendation that you read earlier in this chapter on fiber should help keep your cholesterol and triglycerides under control. Take into consideration once again that we are against fat-free diets because cholesterol and fats are needed for the growing fetus. If you don't eat enough fat, your body may produce its own cholesterol.

GESTATIONAL DIABETES

A week doesn't go by without our seeing a newly diagnosed pregnant woman with gestational diabetes. The basic goal is to restrict simple sugars in the diet and eat at regular intervals. Some ideas are listed below followed by a sample meal plan. If you are told you have gestational diabetes, we recommend that you consult with a dietitian to develop a plan specifically for you. The dietitian can help incorporate many of the foods you like as well as help you plan for special occasions.

- Avoid juice whether you have diabetes or not. The sugar in juice is a simple one and is absorbed readily. It is also high in calories.
- Avoid milk in the morning because of the lactose (milk sugar). Glucose tolerance—the way your body handles sugar—is the worst in the morning. For that reason, skip cereal and milk in the morning and have it as a nighttime snack.
- Eat three meals and three snacks per day instead of the usual three large meals. This is a good way for your body

to become accustomed to utilizing calories throughout the day instead of concentrating them into one or two big meals.

- Always include a protein with the carbohydrates that you eat at your meals and snacks.
- Try to avoid all candy, cookies, and cakes.
- Follow the sample meal plans listed on the next few pages. If you don't drink the milk listed, you can substitute some low-fat cheese or an additional ounce of low-fat meat (chicken, turkey, or low-fat beef).

How to Adjust the Calorie Level of Your Meal Plan

We call these our simple math menus because if you are gaining too fast or not gaining enough, you can add or subtract 200 calories in either direction by using the food blocks below. Because you have gestational diabetes, do not add your extra calories in the form of fruit or sugar. If you are really hungry in the morning, speak to your dietitian or diabetes educator about what you can safely add to the morning meal and/or snack. Eliminate or add foods in the following manner:

☐ 1 starch (80 calories)
☐ 1 meat (55–100 calories)
☐ 1 fat (45 calories)
☐ 1 vegetable (25 calories)

If your goal is to gain more weight, keep the number of servings per block the same but choose foods from the B or C blocks. If you need to reduce your intake, choose primarily A-block foods.

Menu 1—2,200 Calories—Gestational Diabetes

Breakfast

1 STARCH:	1/2 whole wheat English muffin
1 MEAT:	1 egg or 2 egg whites
VEGETABLES:	mushrooms, onions (to scramble with egg)
2 FATS:	2 t. butter, margarine, or oil

Midmorning Snack

1 STARCH	2 rice cakes (any variety)
1/2 MEAT:	1 T. natural peanut or almond butter

Lunch

2 STARCHES:	2 slices whole-wheat bread or whole pita
3 MEATS:	3 oz grilled chicken breast
VEGETABLES:	tomatoes, lettuce
1 FRUIT:	1 pear
2 FATS:	2 t. regular mayo, 2 T. light mayo, or 1/4 avocado
1/2 MILK:	4 oz nonfat or 1 percent milk

Midafternoon Snack (the sticks)

2 STARCHES:	1 1/2 ounce pretzel sticks (whole wheat)
2 MEATS:	2 oz low-fat string cheese
VEGETABLE:	any "sticks" (carrot, jicama, cucumber, zucchini)
1 FAT:	2 T. light dressing (for dipping)

Dinner

2 STARCHES:	2/3 cup brown rice (steamed in chicken or vegetable broth)
3 MEATS:	3 oz lean, broiled steak (like small filet)
VEGETABLES:	steamed broccoli or cauliflower
1 FRUIT:	baked apple or 1/2 cup natural applesauce
2 FATS:	2 t. olive oil or butter (use on vegetables or salad)
1/2 MILK:	4 oz nonfat or 1 percent milk

Evening Snack:

2 STARCHES	4 Wasa crackers
1/2 MEAT:	1 T. peanut or almond butter
1/2 MILK:	4 oz nonfat or 1 percent milk

Menu 2—2,200 Calories—Gestational Diabetes

Breakfast

1 STARCH:	1 slice whole-wheat bread
1 MEATS:	¼ cup cottage cheese topped with cinnamon (optional)
2 FATS:	12 chopped roasted almonds or cashews

Midmorning Snack

1 STARCH:	1 mini whole-wheat bagel
½ MEAT:	1 T. peanut, almond, or soy butter

Lunch

2 STARCHES:	2 slices whole-wheat bread or whole pita
3 MEATS:	3 oz sliced turkey breast
VEGETABLES:	tomatoes, lettuce
1 FRUIT:	2 small tangerines
1 FAT:	2 t. regular mayo, 1 T. light mayo, or ¼ avocado
½ MILK:	4 oz nonfat or 1 percent milk

Midafternoon Snack:

2 STARCH:	1 whole wheat tortilla (approx. 160 calories)
2 MEATS:	2 oz low fat cheese
1 FRUIT:	2 small tangerines
1 FAT:	⅛ avocado combined with salsa

Dinner (Burger night)

2 STARCHES:	1 whole wheat bun
3 MEATS:	3 oz lean ground beef, turkey, chicken, fish, or vegetable patty
VEGETABLES:	lettuce, tomato, onion (for burger), and small green salad
2 FATS:	2 T. light mayonnaise or 2 T. light dressing
1 FRUIT:	1 cup berries (okay to blend with milk for smoothie)
½ MILK:	4 oz nonfat or 1 percent milk (+ add 1 cup ice cubes to blender)

Evening Snack:

2 STARCH:	6 cups popcorn (microwave (light) or air-popped)
1 MEAT:	1 oz cheese
1 FAT:	1 t. butter for popcorn
½ MILK:	½ cup nonfat or 1 percent plain yogurt

Menu 3—2,200 Calories—Gestational Diabetes

Breakfast

1 STARCH:	1/2 cup oatmeal
1 MEAT:	1/4 cup cottage cheese
1 FAT:	1 t. butter

Mid-morning Snack (quesadilla snack)

1 STARCH:	1 corn tortilla
1 MEAT:	1 oz light cheese, melted
1 FAT:	1/8 avocado (okay to add chopped tomato or salsa)

Lunch

2 STARCHES:	2 slices whole-wheat bread or whole pita
3 MEATS:	3/4 cup canned, water packed tuna or salmon
VEGETABLES:	tomatoes, lettuce
1 FRUIT:	17 small grapes or 1 dozen larger grapes
1 FAT:	2 t. regular mayo, 1 T. light mayo, or 1/4 avocado
1/2 MILK:	4 oz nonfat or 1 percent milk

Midafternoon Snack:

2 STARCHES:	low-fat wheat crackers that equal 160 calories per serving
2 MEATS:	1 whole egg and 2 whites, hard-boiled for egg salad
1 FRUIT:	1/2 banana
1 FAT:	1 T. low-fat mayonnaise (for egg salad)

Dinner (Asian delight)

2 STARCHES:	1 cup noodles or 2/3 cup rice (try brown rice)
4 MEATS:	4 oz lean beef or chicken strips, stir-fried (see fat)
VEGETABLES:	assorted peppers, onion, bean sprouts, and carrots
1 FRUIT:	1/2 cup canned mandarin oranges or 2 small tangerines
1 FAT:	1 t. peanut or sesame oil for stir-frying

Evening Snack:

1 MEAT:	1 oz low-fat string cheese
1/2 MILK:	4 oz nonfat or 1 percent milk
1 BREAD:	1/2 cup shredded-wheat-and-bran cereal
2 FATS:	12 almonds or cashews

Menu 4—2,200 Calories—Gestational Diabetes

Breakfast (it's hot!)

1 STARCHES:	½ cup Cream of Wheat or grits (measure ½ cup after cooking)
2 FATS:	6 chopped roasted almonds and 1 t. butter or margarine
1 MEAT:	1 egg (any style)

Midmorning Snack

1 BREAD:	2 popcorn cakes
½ MEAT:	1 T. peanut, almond, or soy butter

Lunch

2 STARCHES:	1 medium baked potato or yam
3 MEATS:	¾ cup cottage cheese or vegetarian chili
VEGETABLES:	broccoli, green onions, and tomato salsa
1 FRUIT:	1 cup honeydew melon
1 FAT:	1 t. butter or margarine or 3 T. light sour cream
½ MILK:	4 oz nonfat, 1 percent milk, or 1 oz shredded light cheese (for potato)

Midafternoon Snack: (PB and banana)

2 STARCHES:	2 slices whole-wheat bread
1 MEAT:	2 T. peanut or almond butter
1 FRUIT:	½ banana

Dinner (Italian night)

2 STARCHES:	1 cup pasta (with fresh tomato-basil sauce)
3 MEATS:	3 oz poached salmon or other allowed fish
VEGETABLES:	fresh salad + broccoli
1 FRUIT:	⅓ cantaloupe
2 FAT:	2 t. olive oil (for pasta or to sauté garlic) or 4 T. light dressing
½ MILK:	4 oz nonfat or 1 percent milk or 1–2 T. grated Parmesan cheese for pasta

Evening Snack:

2 STARCHES	6 cups popcorn (microwave (light) or air-popped)
1 MEAT	1 oz low-fat cheese
½ MILK	4 oz nonfat or 1 percent
2 FATS	2 t. butter or margarine

Laurie's Story

In anticipation of becoming pregnant, Laurie had been attending weekly sessions with a weight-loss group. Her starting weight was 230 pounds. She wanted to get below 200 pounds before getting pregnant. She had begun to eat healthfully for the first time in her life. She had been losing weight at the rate of two to three pounds a week. She had gotten pregnant in January and then miscarried in March. Her weight two weeks after she miscarried was 210 pounds. Her physician advised her to try to avoid getting pregnant for the next three months. Because she had been distraught about the loss of the fetus, Laurie did not resume her dietary restrictions. She remembered being told that dieting is not recommended during pregnancy. Thinking that she would be pregnant soon, she decided not to cut back on her food intake.

Laurie did get pregnant by June, but had not lost the 10 pounds that she had put on prior to the miscarriage in January. A certified public accountant, Laurie had just finished overworking during tax season. Because she had to spend many late nights and weekends at work, her company ordered dinner in. She was not in charge of the food choices. She had to forgo the daily walks with her husband and puppy. What was she to do now?

Laurie's Current Profile
"The Facts"
- Prepregnant weight: 210 pounds
- Current weight: 222 pounds
- Height: 5 feet 6 inches
- Goal for weight gain in pregnancy: 15–25 pounds
- Number of weeks pregnant: 15
- Total weight gain: 12 pounds

At fifteen weeks of pregnancy, Laurie had gained almost 12 pounds. Because her weight-gain goal for the entire pregnancy was 15 to 25 pounds, her doctor referred her to our office for medical nutrition therapy. She had been told to gain one-half to three-quarters of a pound a week, but had gained 8 pounds the past month. In the first eleven weeks of pregnancy she had gained 4 pounds. She felt that she was on the right track. What happened during this last month?

A look at her food diary showed that she had been drinking three, 8-ounce glasses of calcium-fortified orange juice per day because she did not drink plain milk. Each morning on the way to work she bought a 16-ounce fat-free decaffeinated mocha and had a low-fat scone. For lunch, she usually ate at the salad bar, thinking that was the better choice than the burgers she'd eaten before losing weight. Dinners were usually cooked at home and were quite well balanced except when Laurie's office brought in food for late-night work sessions. She had substituted regular lemon-lime soda for the diet cola she had been drinking prior to getting pregnant. She had been unable to take her daily walks.

RECOMMENDATIONS FOR LAURIE

Calcium fortified orange juice: Laurie should start taking calcium pills and skip the juice. Eat three to four fruits a day rather than an amount of juice that equals six fruits.

Fat-free latte: Thinking that a fat-free mocha was harmless because it did not contain fat, she ordered one daily. What she didn't realize was that it contained approximately 250 calories. The recommendation was to order a small latte or decaffeinated coffee with nonfat milk.

Low-fat scone: The scone, though low-fat, was quite large and equivalent to eating approximately four slices of bread. We put it on a food scale, and indeed it weighed four-plus ounces. Laurie decided that eating plain oatmeal at breakfast with fresh fruit was a better choice.

Salad bar: The only recommendation regarding the salad bar was for Laurie to put the dressing in a small container on the side instead of on the salad. This way she could "dip" the salad into the dressing instead of pouring it over the top. She could save several hundred calories by doing this.

Lemon-lime soda: Laurie's idea of giving up the diet drinks was a good one, but replacing them with a can of soda that had 150 calories (equivalent to nine teaspoons of sugar) was not the best beverage choice. She agreed to start drinking water or decaffeinated iced tea.

Late-night dinners at the office: When ordering Asian food, get it steamed instead of stir-fried. Steamed brown or white rice is better than fried rice. Brown rice has the benefit of added fiber. Laurie learned it was best to order her own portion instead of sharing with her office mates.

Inability to exercise: Laurie agreed to ride an exercycle when watching the news in the morning or talking on the phone in the evening. For the time being, this could take the place of walking the puppy.

Other Tips for Laurie

- If bringing food from home, pack lunches according the nutrition plan. If dining out, select a menu that resembles her meal plan as closely as possible. For example:

  Lunch A: turkey sandwich, small vegetable salad, one cup fruit salad

  Lunch B: grilled fish, baked potato, steamed vegetables, berries

- Keep a daily food diary and check in with the dietitian every two weeks.
- Keep a water bottle under her desk to drink instead of soda if she gets thirsty at the office.
- Pack a cooler with healthy snacks (see chapter 13).

Final Outcome

Weight gain began to taper off to one-half to three-quarters of a pound per week. The baby was born two weeks early. The total weight gain had been 30 pounds. The baby weighed 7 pounds 7 ounces. We considered this a successful outcome.

Chapter Thirteen

Eating on the Go as You Grow

One of the most important tips that we hope you get from reading this book is learning to plan meals for yourself. We feel that this is the key to keeping your weight under control during and after pregnancy. Most people tend to make poor food choices when they are overly hungry and look for the quickest thing to eat. Unfortunately, quick foods are usually high in calories and fat but low in nutritional value. In this chapter, we will tell you what you need to know in order to make good food choices when you find yourself on the go and hungry.

Fast Foods Don't Have to Be Bad Foods

Luckily, there are many healthy and tasty selections to choose among when you are tired, lazy, or too busy to prepare dinner. If you can't always afford the time (or money) to dine out in a classy manner, there are some good and economical alternatives to preparing home-cooked meals. Start by looking at your food plan. Make your selections match what you should be eating as closely as possible. Many fast-food establishments provide menus with nutritional information on the Web, on their premises, or even at their drive-through windows.

Eating fast food occasionally is okay as long as you are aware of the following pitfalls:

- Some meals might not contain adequate vitamins, minerals, and calcium. (Try to order skim milk as your beverage and order salads and vegetables if they are available.)

- Sandwiches are usually made with white bread. (When available, select whole wheat).

- Some choices may be higher in fat. (Don't let them grill the bun or add mayonnaise.)

- Beverages are high in calories. (Select water or milk as your first option. Avoid punch, regular soda, and lemonade. If you must have something sweet, mix one-third lemonade to two-thirds water.)

- Most fast foods are low in folic acid because they rarely contain vegetables. (Add vegetables later in the day as a snack.)

- If you have to watch your salt intake, check the nutrition facts available at most fast-food restaurants and make your selections wisely.

For all the above reasons, it is okay to eat fast foods occasionally, but make sure you also include some home-cooked meals in your diet as well.

Our Favorite Fast-Food Ideas

■ Submarine sandwiches: Choose turkey, roast beef, or veggie. Hold the extra mayonnaise and oil unless you put it on yourself.

■ Burger option #1: Choose the grilled or broiled chicken sandwich, hold the sauce, and add ketchup or mustard with the lettuce and tomato. (Hint: Ask for your bun "dry." Because of the fat on the grill, do not let them grill it.)

■ Burger option #2: If you feel like beef, choose the small hamburger (no added mayo or sauce).

■ French fries: If you feel a craving for fries, order the small size or ask for a half-size portion. If they refuse, offer the extra fries to a friend or throw them away before you start eating.

■ Salads: Chopped vegetable or grilled chicken salad are always good choices. Always ask for dressing on the side.

■ Dressings: Vinaigrette is always best. Stay away from thick, mayonnaise-based dressings.

■ Chinese quickies: Steamed white or brown rice, with steamed vegetables and chicken or shrimp. Even though the flavored chicken is great, if it is deep-fried, it's not great for you. Order a plain dish and ask for sweet-and-sour sauce on the side.

■ Mexican: Soft chicken or grilled fish (not fried) tacos, boiled beans, and chicken or vegetable fajitas can be ordered with less oil. Avoid refried beans because they have added fat and sometimes lard. Tostados are fine if you order them without the shell, guacamole, and sour cream. Turn down the chips or count out ten and eat them slowly with salsa.

- Pizza/Italian: One slice of pizza is usually enough, and if you blot the oil off the top before eating, you will reduce the fat. Another option is to order plain pasta, with marinara sauce. Skip the garlic bread but round out the meal with a salad.

- Baked potato bar: Top off your potato with steamed vegetables. Lightly sprinkle with cheese. Avoid sour cream and cheese sauce (unless they are low fat) but try some salsa or cottage cheese instead.

- Teriyaki bowls: Go for the grilled chicken, steamed brown or white rice, and steamed vegetables. If the portion of rice is large, ask for less rice and more vegetables. Other options besides chicken are shrimp, fish, or lean beef. Order the teriyaki sauce on the side so that you control how much you use.

HEALTHY "QUICK" FOOD IDEAS FOR BREAKFAST

- Toasted English muffin and scrambled eggs
- Egg white omelet with half a bagel and jelly (no cream cheese)
- Oatmeal with a quarter cup of raisins and skim milk
- High-fiber breakfast cereal with milk and fruit
- Whole-wheat bread with cottage cheese and cinnamon

RESTAURANT LUNCH AND DINNER TIPS

If you need to entertain a client or attend a business lunch or dinner, what should you select? Think healthy by slimming down your menu choices.

	Choose	Skip
Protein	Grilled chicken or fish	Heavy sauces on entrée
	Grilled chicken sandwich	Cheeseburger
Vegetable	Salads (dressing on side)	Salads tossed with dressing
Bread	Slice of bread (no butter)	Croutons
Starch	Baked Potato	Mashed or fried
Vegetables	Steamed or grilled	Tempura, sautéed, or creamed
Fruit	Any fresh fruit	Fruit pie
Beverage	Water or decaf iced tea	Regular soda or lemonade

OUR BEST DINING TIPS

- Skip the olive oil and butter served with bread.
- Ask for the bun to be toasted instead of grilled.
- No mayonnaise added to your sandwich unless you do it!
- Substitute chicken in your chopped salad for salami and cheese.
- Choose mozzarella, when available, over such other cheeses as Cheddar and American.
- Order Asian foods steamed instead of stir-fried.
- Order a tostado without the fried shell, get soft tortillas on the side instead.
- Never add cheese to your sandwich if it already includes a source of protein (unless you need more calcium in your diet).
- If you have ordered a grilled vegetable sandwich, do add the cheese.
- If fats and oils are being used in the meal preparation, ask the waiter to have your order made with less oil.

Munchies and Vending Machines

Do you have a vending machine near your office? Quite often they contain sandwiches, yogurt, cottage cheese, and fresh fruit. Refer to your nutrition plan to see where these foods fit in. For snacks, select the yogurt, pretzels, animal crackers, baked chips, raisins, and healthier-looking trail mix. Some vending machines even indicate the healthier choices. Keep the intake of these foods in moderation. If you select six nuts, it is the same as eating a teaspoon of oil on your salad. If the package comes with thirty nuts, take what you are allowed and save the rest for later or share them with a coworker or friend. Drink water or herbal tea to keep you hydrated and quench your thirst. Regular gum contains sugar, so chew it in moderation. If you have gestational diabetes, you should choose sugarless gum. Since this type of gum is artificially sweetened, you should limit its use.

BE YOUR OWN VENDOR

Another option is to be your own vending machine. This will not only be cost-effective, but you'll have healthy snacks at your fingertips, all day. Whether you are on the road or at the office, your cooler can be your vending machine. Here are some foods to consider putting in your cooler:

- Baby carrots, grape tomatoes, and/or sliced vegetables
- Four-ounce yogurts
- Sliced oranges or other fresh fruits
- A sandwich for lunch or cut in quarters for snacks
- Low-fat string cheese or other light cheeses
- Pretzel sticks, whole-wheat crackers, or mini rice cakes
- Popcorn (light, air-popped)

Pack your "vending cooler" when you put your food away after dinner. If you do this at night, it doesn't become something extra you need to do in the morning. Hopefully, your cooler will have enough choices to avoid feeling tempted when you walk past the vending machine or the chocolate on someone's desk.

SOME MORE SNACK CHOICES

Give me something sweet, give me something I like to eat!

Don't be surprised if you need to send you husband or significant other out for something sweet at a moment's notice. Just hand him this list of healthy snacks so that you can make good choices. Here are some of our favorites that are about 80 to 100 calories per serving.

- ☐ 7 animal crackers
- ☐ 4 dried apricots
- ☐ 3 graham cracker squares (any flavor)
- ☐ ¾ oz of pretzels
- ☐ 1 baby box of raisins
- ☐ 3 cups light popcorn
- ☐ Snack-size can of fruit in its own juice
- ☐ 1 frozen-fruit bar
- ☐ ⅓ cup hummus with vegetable sticks
- ☐ 4–5 low-fat meringue cookies
- ☐ 2 large flavored rice cakes
- ☐ 2 large flavored corn cakes

☐ 2 peanut-butter-and-cheese sandwich crackers

☐ 10 pistachio nuts

☐ ¾ cup cereal and milk

☐ 1 oz baked chips

☐ ½ cup sorbet

☐ 1 cup soup (noncream)

☐ 1 cup fresh fruits or berries

☐ 1 mini crisp rice/marshmallow bar (.78 oz)

☐ 1 packet of hot cocoa

☐ 4–6 low-fat wheat crackers

☐ 4 small Tootsie Rolls (if you have a craving for sweets)

Reading Labels

When you look at the information on food labels, the percent daily value on the right side of the label is usually based on a 2,000-calorie diet. This is close to what you will be eating, so you can feel free to use it as a basis for comparing one product with another. Overall, learning to read food labels is one of the most important things you can do to improve what you eat. Labels tell you what the food is composed of and therefore allow you to make informed choices.

The first thing you should look at on any food label is the "number of servings per package." For example, if you see a muffin label that says the calories in one serving are 150 but find out that there are four servings in the package, the calories in the whole muffin would be 600! Who needs that?

When looking at a box of cereal, you should pay attention to the calories and how much is considered one serving. Below are two cereals to compare.

	Shredded Wheat and Bran	Low-fat Granola with Raisins
Serving size:	1¼ cups	⅔ cup
Calories	200	210
Fat	1 gram	3 grams
Fiber	8 grams	3 grams
Sodium	0 mg	130 mg
Protein	7 grams	4 grams

In the above example, note that the number of calories in both cereals are similar, but you are getting a larger portion and more fiber when you choose the shredded wheat and bran! Doing this kind of comparison when selecting breads, crackers, soups, frozen products, cookies, and other foods will help you make good choices.

Frozen/TV Dinners

Sometimes it may be necessary to have some frozen dinners on hand at work or home in order to avoid eating without planning. These can come in handy if you are too sick, too lazy, or too busy to cook. We usually don't recommend these as a steady diet, but once in a while you'll be glad you have them in your freezer. Evaluate the products by reading the label. Doing some comparison shopping among brands will give you an idea of which ones to choose. Basically, for one portion you should use these guidelines:

- Protein level should be about 21 grams or higher per serving. (If less than 14 grams, you should add an extra ounce of protein to your meal—such as low-fat shredded cheese, cottage cheese, or a half cup of beans.)

- Fat should be limited to 10 grams or less.

- Sodium levels can vary; try to choose a product that is between 600 and 1000 milligrams.

- Calorie levels should be around 300 to 400. Use the frozen dinner as the basis of your meal and round it out with a fresh vegetable salad, fruit, and a glass of milk.

One final suggestion is to consider making your own frozen meals with leftovers. You can "throw in" leftover meat, vegetables, and pasta and freeze them in the great new disposable containers available in the market.

The Overrated "Health" Food—Juices, Smoothies, and Blended Drinks

Most people think that juices and smoothies are healthy. Yes, they are healthy if you need to gain weight. Are you aware that most smoothies at juice bars have between 400 and 700 calories per drink? This can be almost a third of your total calories for the day! These drinks are high in simple sugars and can be low in fiber. If the drink is "clear," you know that it has little fiber. Most of the fiber from these blended juices ends up in the garbage, and unfortunately that is the part that would be the most healthy and filling for you. Our motto is keep the fruit in its original package and you'll be doing yourself a favor! Also, don't drink the "ades" such as lemonade or limeade. They will also add empty calories and not "aid" in keeping your weight under control in this pregnancy. Lemonade is *not* lemon juice. It takes about nine to twelve packages of sugar to sweeten one glass of lemonade.

In the event that you are experiencing morning sickness and all you can tolerate is juice, then blend your own smoothie with fresh fruit and skim milk or yogurt.

Some other ways to enjoy juice is to spoon one or two tablespoons of juice over your freshly prepared fruit salad to help sweeten it and keep it from turning brown. Remember, there are often as many calories in juice as in the same portion of soda. That is why juice is not really a healthy alternative to soda. If you're worried about not getting the vitamins in juice, choose whole fruits, which have the vitamins plus all-important fiber.

Below you will find a "juice chart" that compares the calories in your favorite juices or juice drinks with alternatives that are lower in calories and may contain the added benefit of fiber.

To Juice or Not to Juice?

Juice and Juice Beverages	Whole Fruit or Vegetable
12 oz orange juice (180 calories)	1 orange (60 calories)
12 oz cranberry/apple drink* (227 calories)	1 small apple (60 calories)
12 oz cranberry juice cocktail* (194 calories)	17 grapes (60 calories)
12 oz grapefruit juice (133 calories)	½ grapefruit (60 calories)
12 oz apple juice (159 calories)	1 small apple (60 calories)
12 oz tangerine juice (169 calories)	2 small tangerines (60 calories)
12 oz juice punch drink* (159 calories)	1¼ cup watermelon (60 calories)

Juice and Juice Beverages	Whole Fruit or Vegetable
12 oz carrot juice (136 calories)	1 cup carrot sticks (25 calories)
12 oz lemonade* (136 calories)	12 oz iced tea/lemon (0 calories)

*These "juice" drinks contain added sugar and are not pure juices.

Blended Coffee Drinks

We wish the news on blended coffee drinks was better than the news on blended juices, but unfortunately the story is the same, if not worse: At least with the juices you get vitamins. Many of these popular drinks contain over 250 calories *before* the whipped cream is added. While coffee has no calories, adding sugar, flavored powders, chocolate, half-and-half, and whipped cream may push the scale upward at your next doctor visit. There is only one time that we recommend having blended coffee drinks and that is during periods of severe morning sickness when you are too nauseous to eat anything else. If this is all you can tolerate, start with decaffeinated coffee and request nonfat milk. One other option is to blend your own decaffeinated coffee drink at home. This way you can control the amount of sugar and the type of milk.

Holiday Tips

Considering the fact that you will be pregnant for nine months, chances are pretty good that you will be celebrating at least one holiday, a birthday, or another special occasion during this time. Celebrations are part of life, and therefore learning how to eat during them is important even when you are not carrying a baby. Here are some of our favorite special occasion/holiday tips.

■ Continue to eat a well-balanced diet.

■ Don't go to a party hungry; always have a light snack before you go.

■ Fill your plate with plenty of vegetables (make vegetables your appetizer of choice instead of the mini "fried" eggrolls, wontons, and hot dogs).

■ Use dips and guacamole in moderation. Dip your vegetables in salsa instead.

■ Eat half portions of such favorite holiday goodies as stuffing, mashed potatoes, yams with marshmallows, gravy, and crescent rolls. You can also pick your favorite and skip the rest. Remember, there will always be another holiday.

■ If you're the cook, send the "dangerous" leftovers home with your guests. (Do this even though sending home the chocolate cake may bring tears to your eyes.)

■ Buffets require special consideration because they can trigger overeating. The first step is to take a trip around the buffet to "check out the scene" and see what appeals to you the most. Start with a salad or a noncream soup and follow it with *one* entrée, starch, and as many steamed or grilled vegetables as your heart desires. For dessert, start with fresh fruit and complete your meal with a small serving of the dessert that you want the most.

■ Skip the alcohol at all parties and events.

■ Drink plenty of fluids such as water, caffeine-free or herbal iced tea, mineral water, or the lowest-fat milk available. Skip the high-calorie juices and eggnogs.

- Don't let other people sabotage your food choices. They may encourage you to eat so they won't feel guilty. Remember, you are in charge of what you eat!

- Birthday cake or your baby-shower cake is part of life. Enjoy a slice but choose a piece from the middle (without excess frosting). Always request a small slice and eat it slowly so that you can enjoy it.

- Share any gift baskets or candy you receive with coworkers or friends. Resist the temptation to take these home. Realize that if you bring them home, you will eat them. (Tell your husband or significant other to do the same thing.)

- Keep active. If your doctor allows you to exercise, keep your program going during the holidays.

- Walk away from the 50-percent-off candy sale after all holidays. Remember the calories are not 50 percent off!

Chapter Fourteen

Breast-feeding: Every Body Benefits

t's the first time I felt like a mom," stated Marlene's niece Stacey. Many new moms realize that breast-feeding can be one of the most pleasurable aspects of having a new baby. Being a nursing mom requires you to spend relaxing moments with your newborn and gives you an opportunity to truly bond. If you are craving quiet time away from friends and family, it's a good excuse to "get away from it all."

You will find that everyone around you has a different opinion about breast-feeding. If your friends and family didn't breast-feed, they may try to discourage you. If they did breast-feed, they will probably encourage you. Many women who had children during the 1940s and 1950s were discouraged from breast-feeding but have since learned of its benefits from their daughters.

The Benefits to Mom

There are many advantages to breast-feeding but one of the best is that you may experience weight loss without much effort. Hopefully, if you are not eating hot fudge sundaes on a nightly basis, this may be the first time in your life that you will reap the benefit of painless weight loss. Once the baby is six weeks old, exercise can become part of your daily routine. Many mothers report that they returned to close to their normal weight within six months. Many women who carried extra weight before pregnancy find they are below that weight after a few months of breast-feeding. A good rate of weight loss is one to two pounds per week. In the first few weeks following delivery, you will lose more weight from the birth of the baby, placenta, and other fluids. After that, you should settle into a pattern of losing more gradually.

If you continue to follow the guidelines in this book, you might also experience the weight-loss benefit of breast-feeding. If you find yourself below your prepregnancy weight, it is fine as long as the baby is gaining the appropriate amount of weight. If this is happening, you can continue to follow the pregnancy meal plan. The fluid requirement is greater but doesn't need to be fulfilled with high calorie drinks. If you are getting enough calcium from cheese or calcium supplements, water is just fine.

In addition to the weight-loss benefit of breast-feeding, there are savings of time and money. You will save plenty of time by not having to prepare and wash bottles and nipples. If you are supplementing with formula, which is expensive, you will clearly see the cost benefit of breast-feeding and be happy you made the decision to breast-feed.

The Benefit to Baby

The nutritional content of human milk is designed especially for your baby, so why not choose your own milk as your babies first food? Here are some of the reasons why breast milk is best for your newborn:

- Breast milk is easier for the baby to digest.

- Baby has less chance for allergies in the future.

- Babies are rarely allergic to Mom's milk but often have allergies to formula.

- Baby is less likely to be overfed and therefore overweight. (Baby will take in only what's needed and Mom has less of a chance to force-feed.)

- There is less chance of contamination from bottles and nipples.

- Baby gets natural immunities from colostrum, the fluid that is produced before the milk arrives.

What to Eat While You're Nursing

The most important rule about what to eat while breast-feeding is never to cut back to less than 1,800 calories per day. This is no time to crash-diet. Producing milk requires additional calories, and if you don't take in those calories, your milk supply may not be adequate. A recent patient of ours started dieting after her baby was born, and as a result, the baby failed to gain the appropriate weight. After reviewing the food diary of the patient, we discovered that she was not getting enough calories.

Once she started to eat more, her milk was in greater supply and the baby started to gain appropriately.

Most nursing moms do well by following the basic pregnancy meal plan outlined in chapter 9. To provide the extra calories needed for nursing, we recommend adding an extra 200 calories per day to your diet. Use this as a baseline, and as long as your baby is gaining enough weight and you are not losing more than two pounds per week, you can safely continue eating this amount. If you provide the calories in the form of two extra glasses milk (nonfat or low-fat), you are getting the added benefit of extra fluid, calcium, protein, vitamins, and minerals.

Other Important Tips for Breast-feeding Moms

- Every time you nurse, drink a glass or water or milk to replenish the fluids used to produce your milk.

- Have your drinks sitting by your side. As your breast milk lets down, you will be extremely thirsty.

- Continue to take your prenatal vitamin even if you feel you are eating a healthy diet.

- Avoid foods that tend to cause you gastrointestinal upset or make your baby particularly irritable. These foods can include broccoli, cabbage, garlic, cauliflower, and onions.

- Caffeine, alcohol, and sugar substitutes should not be used, as they are passed along to the baby through your breast milk.

- Chocolate and other foods that contain caffeine should be used only in moderation. (See chapter 8 for list of caffeine-containing foods.)

▪ Always check with your doctor before taking over-the-counter medications or other medications prescribed by another doctor.

What to Eat After Nursing (or If You Decided Not to Nurse)

A well-balanced diet and adequate vitamin and calcium intake are still important after you stop nursing. The 1,600-calorie sample menu listed below is a basic guide; it is one you can follow, but it has not been designed *specifically* for you. For that reason, this might be a good time to see a registered dietitian, who can provide you with the support and education that you need for your new role as a healthy, fit mom. Special foods that you like can be incorporated into a healthy meal plan. Once you've carried a baby, delivered it, possibly breast-fed an infant, and lost some of your prepregnant weight, you will have a head start should you become pregnant again.

Use the food blocks in chapter 9 to choose your healthy 1,600-calorie diet.

How to Adjust the Calorie Level of Your Meal Plan

If you remember from previous chapters, we call these our simple math menus because if you are gaining too fast or not gaining enough, you can add or subtract 200 calories by using the food blocks below. Eliminate or add foods in the following manner:

1 starch (80 calories)

1 meat (55–100 calories)

1 fat (45 calories)

After-Nursing Sample Menu—1,600 Calories

Breakfast (it's hot!)

2 STARCHES:	1 cup hot oatmeal or Cream of Wheat (measure 1 cup after cooking)
1 FRUIT:	2 T. raisins
1 MILK:	8 oz nonfat or 1 percent milk
1 FAT:	6 chopped roasted almonds or 1 t. butter or margarine

Midmorning Snack

1 FRUIT:	sliced fresh apple

Lunch

2 STARCHES:	1 medium baked potato or yam
3 MEATS:	3/4 cup cottage cheese or 3/4 cup vegetarian chili or 1 chicken breast
VEGETABLES:	broccoli, green onions, and tomato salsa
1 FRUIT:	1 cup honeydew melon
1 FAT:	1 t. butter or margarine or 3 T. light sour cream

Midafternoon Snack

VEGETABLE:	Vegetable sticks with nonfat dressing or salsa

Dinner (Italian night)

2 STARCHES:	1 cup pasta or 2/3 cup brown rice
4 MEATS:	4 oz poached salmon or other A-block protein foods
VEGETABLES:	fresh broccoli, assorted salad greens
1 FRUIT:	1/3 cantaloupe
2 FATS:	2 t. olive oil (for pasta or to sauté garlic) or 4 T. light dressing
FREE:	nonfat salad dressing, lemon juice, or balsamic vinegar

Evening Snack

1 STARCH:	3 graham cracker squares or 1/2 cup bran cereal
1 MILK:	8 oz nonfat or 1 percent milk or 8 oz light yogurt

Take off or add the above to any meal during the day. If you need additional calories, you can add a snack or simply eat more food at one meal.

Chapter Fifteen

The Bottom Line

I n the previous chapters we have summarized much of the research on obesity, fertility, pregnancy, and nutrition to help you become knowledgeable and prepared for a healthy pregnancy. This chapter summarizes the take-home messages and answers some of the most common questions.

- Body Mass Index or BMI relates weight to height and is used by health professionals to define normal weight, underweight, overweight, and obesity. If your BMI is between 25 and 29.9, you are considered overweight. The definition of obesity is a BMI greater than 30.

- The susceptibility to obesity is controlled by our genetics in a complex pattern that has yet to be unraveled. Our environment also plays a role. Our species was designed to be efficient at using energy and storing fat to survive, and this design can lead to obesity when physical activity decreases and food is easily available.

■ Our bodies appear to have a set point that adjusts both food intake and energy use to maintain a particular body weight. This means that losing and maintaining weight can be very difficult and that overweight may be normal for some individuals.

■ Antiobesity drugs, used long term, may act to change the set point but cannot be used during pregnancy.

■ A small weight loss of 5 to 10 percent in people who are obese can make a major difference in hypertension, diabetes, and overall health.

■ Overweight can affect fertility, causing irregular periods and preventing ovulation. Fortunately either a small weight loss or the use of fertility drugs will usually restore normal ovulation in most women.

■ Dieting during pregnancy is a bad idea because the calories go first to the mother and the baby gets only what is left over. However, overweight women do not need to gain as much weight as thin women to produce a healthy baby. For a woman with a BMI between 26 and 29, a gain of 15 to 25 pounds is adequate. For women with a BMI over 30, the recommended weight gain is a minimum of 15 pounds.

■ Pregnancy complications in overweight women are not correlated with the amount of weight gained. However, women who are overweight or obese at the time they become pregnant do have a higher rate of overall complications.

■ Pregnancy can predispose to obesity later in life.

- Women who are overweight and pregnant are at increased risk for chronic hypertension, pregnancy-induced hypertension, preeclampsia, gestational diabetes, stillbirth, and congenital anomalies.

- Babies of women who are both obese and diabetic at the time of pregnancy have three times the overall risk of having some kind of congenital defect.

- Although some of these complications are not preventable, early diagnosis with excellent prenatal care and management can assure a good outcome.

- Because of the increased complication rate, and an increased incidence of very large babies, overweight women tend to have a higher rate of cesarean-section delivery.

- During the postpartum period, overweight women have a higher incidence of wound infections, uterine infection, and venous blood clots.

- Exercise in pregnancy helps maintain cardiovascular fitness, increases endurance, and prepares women for the athletic event of delivery. Exercise programs for the very overweight woman may need to be modified to avoid cardiac stress.

- Preconceptual planning, good prenatal care, competent nutritional guidance, and early diagnosis can help make your pregnancy and your baby as healthy as possible.

Our Favorite Questions

Q: *Will my child be thinner if I breast-feed?*

A: A lot of factors determine the answer to this question. Some of the variables include the baby's birth weight, the genetics of both parents, and the home environment. Breast-feeding may help control weight because it's thought that the breast-fed baby will take only what he needs. Quite often, parents encourage babies to finish a bottle for fear they will not be getting enough food (or wasting formula). This can set up a pattern of overfeeding.

Q: *Will I lose weight faster if I breast-feed?*

A: One thing that we do know about breast-feeding is that you will be thinner if you choose to breast-feed your baby and don't overeat. You expend energy when you breast-feed. In most cases, women who breast-feed report that weight "melts" off without too much effort.

Q: *I was 80 pounds overweight before I got pregnant. What can I do to keep things under control?*

A: Avoid high-fat or fried foods, high-calorie desserts, drink the lowest fat milk you can tolerate, and drink water instead of soda and juice. Keep a food diary to help you evaluate your food intake. Weigh yourself weekly. If this doesn't work, see a nutrition professional.

Q: *I have lost five pounds in the first trimester because of morning sickness. Is that harmful to my baby?*

A: Unless you are dehydrated, losing weight in the first trimester is not harmful. Many women lose weight during the first few months because of morning sickness. Your doctor can reassure you that this is not a concern. When you do feel better, start adding foods that you can tolerate in small, frequent "meals."

Q: *I can't drink milk. What are my options for calcium?*

A: Many women find it difficult to drink milk when they are pregnant. There are many good options, but if weight gain is excessive, it's best to ask your doctor for a calcium supplement to get the 1200 mg needed daily. Also attempt to drink fortified soy milk or eat nonfat or low-fat cheese.

Q: *I stopped taking my iron pills because I'm constipated. Can I get enough iron from my diet?*

A: A good option to increase your iron is to have a serving of iron-fortified cereals such as Total on a daily basis. You can increase the absorption of the iron by eating an orange or grapefruit (high in vitamin C) with your cereal. When eating leafy greens or beans that are high in iron, also include an additional vitamin-C food at the same meal so that the absorption can be enhanced.

Q: *I'm carrying twins. How much should I gain?*

A: If your doctor feels that you were overweight before conception, you should try to gain about 25 to 35 pounds total.

Q: *My nausea won't go away and I'm in my sixth month. I was told it would go away in a few weeks. Do you have any suggestions?*

A: Our suggestion is to try eating six small meals daily and reduce the amount of liquid you drink with meals. If you can't keep food down and you are continuing to lose weight, your doctor may recommend nutritional supplements or antinausea remedies. Do not take anything on your own.

Q: *I'm a binge eater and find it hard to break the cycle.*

A: Most binge eaters have fewer cravings when the meals they eat are well balanced. Eating every few hours keeps you from focusing on food. Don't allow yourself to become overly hungry because that may trigger a binge.

Q: *Breakfast is hard for me to eat because I leave for work very early. What fast-food ideas do you have?*

A: Prepare a cheese sandwich or peanut-butter-and-banana sandwich before you go to bed. You can always turn the cheese sandwich into a "microwaved melt." If you have the time to eat a bowl of cereal, measure out the appropriate amount the night before.

Q: *Can I diet while I'm breast-feeding?*

A: If you gained the recommended amount of weight while you were pregnant, continue to follow your eating plan while you are breast-feeding. If you do this, you will most likely lose weight at a rate of one to two pounds per week. You can also increase your exercise when your doctor says it is okay to do so. If the weather permits, start taking the baby out for walks in the stroller.

Q: *Can I drink a glass of wine while I'm breast-feeding?*

A: Ask your pediatrician because doctors have different philosophies about this subject.

Q: *I take herbal supplements such as echinacea. Is it safe to use these during the pregnancy and while I breast-feed?*

A: Since herbal supplements are not FDA-regulated, we advise you to avoid them.

Q: *I love to eat the "Sunday restaurant breakfast special" with my family. I usually pick two eggs, two strips of bacon, biscuits, and hash browns. Can I still have these?*

A: We'd love to say have it all, but the best way to eat meals like this is to cut the portion size in half. Ask the server to cut the portions and substitute some fresh fruit for the missing items. You can also share the entire breakfast with a friend or relative.

Q: *Can you recommend some good Web sites about food and food safety?*

A: Here are some of our favorite Web sites.

Tufts Nutrition Navigator
www.navigator.tufts.edu
This Web site rates Internet nutrition information and can provide you with links to the Web sites that its writers feel are useful.

The American Dietetic Association
www.eatright.org
This is the Web site for the nutrition and dietetic association.

National Heart, Lung and Blood Institute of the National Institutes of Health
www.nhlbi.nih.gov
The site gives you guidelines for keeping your heart healthy.

InteliHealth, Inc.
www.intelihealth.com
This site leads you to a wealth of health information.

Food Guide Pyramid
www.nal.usda.gov:8001/py/pmap.htm
This site explains current ideas about how much to eat of what group. It contains a visual guide of food proportions.

Dietary Guidelines for Healthy Americans
www.nal.usda.gov/fnic/dga/dguide
The site discusses principles of healthy eating for all
Americans.

Overeaters Anonymous
www.overeatersanonymous.org
The site for a support group for people with eating disorders
including overeating.

Children's Nutrition Research Center
www.bcm.tmc.edu/cnrc/
This is the site of the USDA research center for nutrient goals
of pregnant women, nursing women, and children.

Food and Drug Administration
www.fda.gov
This site offers information on dietary supplements, additives,
food, and drugs.

American Diabetes Association
www.diabetes.org
This site provides information for all types of diabetes.

Consumer Information Center
www.pueblo.gsa.gov
This site lists many available educational materials to purchase
or order for free. There are also some links to brochures available on the Internet; many have been written or reviewed by
government agencies.

FDA's Food Safety Web Site
www.cfsan.fda.gov

NOTES

Chapter 1

1. Hansen B. Emerging strategies for weight management, *Postgraduate Medicine Special Report* (June 2001): 3–9.
2. Kuczmarski RJ, Flegal KM, Campbell SM, et al. Increasing prevalence of overweight among US adults. The National Health and Nutrition Examination Surveys 1960–1991, *Journal of the American Medical Association* 272:3 (1994): 205–211.
3. Mokdad AH, Serdula MK, Dietz WH, et al. The spread of the obesity epidemic in the United States, 1991–1998, *Journal of the American Medical Association* 282:16 (1999): 1519–1522.
4. National Center for Health Statistics. Prevalence of overweight and obesity among adults: United States 1999. Available at: *http://www.cdc. gov/nchs/products/pubs/pubs/hestats/obese/obese99.htm*.
5. Barsh GS, Farooqu I, et al. Genetics of body-weight regulation, *Nature* 404:6778 (April 2000): 644–651.
6. Maes H, Neale MC, and Eaves LF. Genetic and environmental factors in relative body weight and human adiposity, *Behavioral Genetics* 27 (1997): 325–351.

7. Perusse L, et al. The human obesity gene map: the 1998 update, *Obesity Research* 7 (1999): 111–129.

8. Ravussin E, Borgardus C. Energy expenditure in the obese: is there a thrifty gene? *Infusionstherapie* 17 (1990): 108–112.

9. Flegal KM, et al. The influence of smoking cessation on the prevalence of overweight in the United States. *New England Journal of Medicine* 333 (1995): 1165–1170.

10. Schoeller DA, Bandini LG, Dietz WH. Inaccuracies in self-reported intake identified by comparison with the doubly labeled water method, *Canadian Journal of Physiology and Pharmacology* 68:7 (July 1990): 941–949.

11. Prentice AM, et al. High levels of energy expenditure in obese women, *British Medical Journal Clinical Research Ed.* 292: 6526 (April 1986): 983–987.

12. Bandini LG, Schoeller DA, Dietz WH. Energy expenditure in obese and nonobese adolescents, *Pediatric Research* 27:2 (Feb. 1990): 198–203.

13. Devlin MJ, et al. Obesity: what mental health professionals need to know, *The American Journal of Psychiatry* 157:6 (June 2000): 854–866.

14. Keesey RE, Hirvonen MD. Body weight set-points: determination and adjustment, *Journal of Nutrition* 127:9 (Sept. 1997): 1875s–1883s.

15. Leibel RL, Hirsch J. Diminished energy requirements in reduced-obese patients, *Metabolism* 2 (1984): 164–170.

16. Mantzoros CS. The role of leptin in human obesity and disease: a review of current evidence, *Annals of Internal Medicine* 130:8 (April 1999): 671–680.

17. *Ibid.*

18. *Ibid.*

19. Cummings DE, Weigle DS, et al. Plasma Ghrelin Levels after diet-induced weight loss or gastric bypass surgery, *New England Journal of Medicine* 346 (21) (2002): 1623-1630.

20. Weintraub M. Long-term weight control: the National Heart, Lung and Blood Institute funded multimodal intervention study, *Clinical Pharmacology Therapeutics* 51 (1992): 581–585.

21. Devlin MJ, et al. *The American Journal of Psychiatry*: 854–866.

22. Fernstrom MH. Treating obesity in the family practice setting, *Postgraduate Medicine, A Special Report, Emerging Strategies for Weight Management* (June 2001): 10–18.

23. National Institutes of Health. Clinical guidelines on the identification,

evaluation and treatment of overweight and obesity in adults—the evidence report, *Obesity Research* 6, Supplement 2 (1998): 51–209.

Chapter 2

1. Labhart A. *Clinical Endocrinology, Theory and Practice,* Berlin: Springer-Verlag, 1986, 624–626.

2. Marshall WA, Tanner JM. Puberty. In Davis JA, Dobbing J, eds, *Scientific Foundations of Pediatrics.* London: Heinmann, 1974, 124–151.

3. Parra A, et al. The relationship of plasma gonadotropins and steroid concentrations to body growth in girls, *Acta Endocrinologica* (Copenhagen) 98 (1981): 161.

4. *Harrison's Principles of Internal Medicine,* 11th ed. New York: McGraw-Hill, 1987, 390.

5. *Ibid.*

6. Bates, WG. Body weight control practice as a cause of infertility, *Clinical Obstetrics and Gynecology* 28:3 (1985): 632–642.

7. Pettigrew R. Obesity and female reproductive function, *British Medical Bulletin* 53:2 (1997): 341–358.

8. Norman RJ. Obesity, polycystic ovary syndrome and anovulation—how are they related? *Current Opinion in Obstetrics and Gynecology* 13:3 (2001): 323–327.

9. *Ibid.*

10. Moghetti P, et al. Metformin effects on clinical features, endocrine and metabolic profiles and insulin sensitivity in polycystic ovary syndrome: a randomized, double-blind, placebo-controlled 6-month trial, followed by open, long-term clinical evaluation, *Journal of Clinical Endocrinology and Metabolism* 85 (2000): 139–146.

11. Morin-Papunen LC, et al. Endocrine and metabolic effects of metformin versus ethinyl estradiol-cyproterone acetate in obese women with polycystic ovary syndrome: a randomized study, *Journal of Clinical Endocrinology and Metabolism* 85 (2000): 3161–3168.

12. Pasquali R, et al. Effect of long-term treatment with metformin added to hypocaloric diet on body composition, fat distribution, and androgen and insulin levels in abdominally obese women with and without the polycystic ovary syndrome, *Journal of Clinical Endocrinology and Metabolism* 85 (2000): 2767–2774.

13. Butzow TL, et al. The decrease in luteinizing hormone secretion in

response to weight reduction is inversely related to the severity of insulin resistance in overweight women, *Journal of Clinical Endocrinology and Metabolism* 85:9 (Sept. 2000): 3271–3275.

14. Kiddy DS, et al. Improvement in endocrine and ovarian function during dietary treatment of obese women with polycystic ovary syndrome, *Clinical Endocrinology Oxford* 36 (1992): 105–111.

15. Clark AM, Thornley B, et al. Weight loss in obese infertile women results in improvement in reproductive outcome for all forms of fertility treatment, *Human Reproduction* 13:6 (1998): 1502–1505.

16. Lashen H, et al. Extremes of body mass do not adversely affect the outcome of superovulation and in-vitro fertilization, *Human Reproduction* 14:3 (1999): 712–715.

17. Dechaud H, Ferron G, et al. Obesity and assisted reproduction techniques, *Contraception Fertility Sex* 26:7–8 (1998): 564–567.

18. Pettigrew, R. *British Medical Bulletin* 341–358.

19. Kiddy DS, et al. *Clinical Endocrinology Oxford* 105–111.

20. Fedorcsak P, et al. Obesity is a risk factor for early pregnancy loss after IVF or ICSI, *Acta Obstetrica Gynecologica Scandanavica* 79:1 (Jan. 2000): 43–48.

Chapter 3

1. Institute of Medicine. Subcommittee on Nutritional Status and Weight Gain During Pregnancy, *Nutrition During Pregnancy*. Washington, DC: Academy Press, 1990.

2. Luke B, Hediger ML, Scholl TO. Point of diminishing returns: when does gestational weight gain cease benefiting birthweight and begin adding to maternal obesity?, *Journal of Maternal and Fetal Medicine* 5:4 (July–Aug. 1996): 168–173.

3. Lederman SA, et al. Body fat and water changes during pregnancy in women with different body weight and weight gain, *Obstetrics and Gynecology* 90:4, part 1 (Oct. 1997): 483–488.

4. Edwards LE, et al. Pregnancy complications and birth outcomes in obese and normal-weight women: effects of gestational weight change, *Obstetrics and Gynecology* 87:3 (March 1996): 389–394.

5. Bianco AT, et al. Pregnancy outcome and weight gain recommendations for the morbidly obese woman, *Obstetrics and Gynecology* 91:1 (Jan. 1998): 97–102.

6. Gunderson EP, et al. The relative importance of gestational gain and maternal characteristics associated with the risk of becoming over-

weight after pregnancy, *International Journal of Obesity and Related Metabolic Disorders* 24:12 (Dec. 2000): 1660–1668.

7. Rossner S, Ohlin A. Pregnancy as a risk factor for obesity: lessons from the Stockholm Pregnancy and Weight Development Study, *Obesity Research* 3, supplement 2 (Sept. 1995): 267s–275s.

Chapter 4

1. Baeten JM, Bukusi EA, Lambe M. Pregnancy complications and outcomes among overweight and obese nulliparous women, *American Journal of Public Health* 91:3 (March 2001): 436–440.

2. Michlin R, et al. Maternal obesity and pregnancy outcome, *Israel Medical Association Journal* 2:1 (Jan. 2000): 10–13.

3. Bianco AT, et al. Pregnancy outcome and weight gain recommendations for the morbidly obese woman, *Obstetrics and Gynecology* 91:1 (Jan. 1998): 97–102.

4. Shaw GM, et al. Risk of neural tube defect-affected pregnancies among obese women, *Journal of the American Medical Association* 275:14 (April 1996): 1093–1096.

5. Moore LL, et al. A prospective study of the risk of congenital defects associated with maternal obesity and diabetes mellitus, *Epidemiology* 11:6 (Nov. 2000): 689–694.

6. Tilton Z, et al. Complications and outcome of pregnancy in obese women, *Nutrition* 5 (1989): 95–99.

7. Johnson SR, et al. Maternal obesity and pregnancy, *Surgery Gynecology and Obstetrics* 164 (1987): 431–437.

8. De Divitiis O, et al. Obesity and cardiac function, *Circulation* 64 (1981): 477.

9. Veille JC, Hanson R. Obesity, pregnancy and left ventricular functioning during the third trimester, *American Journal of Obstetrics and Gynecology* 171 (1994): 980.

10. Tomoda S, et al. Effects of obesity on pregnant women: maternal hemodynamic change, *American Journal of Perinatology* 13:2 (Feb. 1996): 73–78.

11. Galtier-Dereure F, Montpeyroux F, et al. Weight excess before pregnancy: complications and cost, *International Journal of Obesity* 19 (1995): 443–448.

12. Isaacs JD, Magann EF, et al. Obstetric challenges of massive obesity complicating pregnancy, *Journal of Perinatology* 14 (1994): 10–14.

13. Sibai BM, Gordon T, et al. The National Institute of Child Health and Human Development Network of Maternal Fetal Medicine Units, Risk factors for preeclampsia in healthy nulliparous women: a prospective multicenter study, *American Journal of Obstetrics and Gynecology* 172 (1995): 642–648.
14. Stone JL, Lockwood CJ, et al. Risk factors for severe preeclampsia, *Obstetrics and Gynecology* 83 (1994): 357–361.
15. Galtier-Dereure F, Montpeyroux F, et al. *International Journal of Obesity,* 443–448.
16. Stone JL, Lockwood CJ, et al. *Obstetrics and Gynecology,* 357–361.
17. Abi-Said D, Annegers JF, et al, Case control study of the risk factors for eclampsia, *American Journal of Epidemiology* 142 (1995): 437–441.
18. Stone JL, Lockwood CJ, et al. *Obstetrics and Gynecology,* 357–361.
19. Schwartz WJ, et al. Blood pressure monitoring during pregnancy: accuracy of portable devices designed for obese patients, *Journal of Reproductive Medicine* 41:8 (1996): 581–585.
20. Cunningham FG, Lowe TW. Cardiovascular Diseases Complicating Pregnancy, Appleton-Century-Crofts, (1991): 2–4. *Williams Obstetrics, 18th ed.*
21. Barton JR, Witlin AG, Sibai BM. Management of mild proeclamsia, *Clinical Obstetrics and Gynecology,* Lippincott Williams and Wilkins, 42:3 (Sept. 1999): 455.
22. American Diabetes Association Position Statement. Gestational diabetes mellitus, *Diabetes Care* 23, supplement 1 (2000).
23. *Ibid.*
24. Kjos SL, Buchanan TA. Current concepts: gestational diabetes mellitus, *New England Journal of Medicine* 341:23 (Dec. 1999): 1749–1756.
25. Leveno KJ, Cunningham F. Gestational Diabetes: Evolving concepts and misconceptions, *Williams Obstetrics,* supplement, 18 ed. Appleton-Century-Crofts, (1986):5.
26. Langer O. Management of gestational diabetes. *Diabetes and Pregnancy, Clinical Obstetrics and Gynecology,* Lippincott Williams and Wilkins, 43:1 (March 2000): 106–115.

Chapter 5

1. Crane SS, Wojtowycz MA, et al. Association between pre-pregnancy obesity and the risk of cesarean delivery, *Obstetrics and Gynecology* 89:2 (1997): 213–216.

2. Kaiser PS, Kirby RS. Obesity as a risk factor for cesarean in a low-risk population, *Obstetrics and Gynecology* 97:1 (Jan. 2001): 39–43.
3. Michlin R, Oettinger M, et al. Maternal obesity and pregnancy outcome, *Israel Medical Association Journal* 2:1 (Jan. 2000): 10–13.
4. Perlow JH, Morgan MA, et al. Perinatal outcome in pregnancy complicated by massive obesity, *American Journal of Obstetrics and Gynecology* 167:4, part 1 (Oct. 1992): 958–962.
5. Isaacs JD, Magann EF, et al. Obstetric challenges of massive obesity complicating pregnancy, *Journal of Perinatology* 14 (1994): 10–14.
6. Perlow JH, Morgan MA. Massive maternal obesity and perioperative cesarean morbidity, *American Journal of Obstetrics and Gynecology* 170:2 (1994): 560–565.
7. Hamza J, et al. Parturient's posture during epidural puncture affects the distance from skin to epidural space, *Journal of Clinical Anesthesia* 7:1 (Feb. 1995): 1–4.
8. *Ibid.*
9. Hood DD, Dewan DM. Anesthetic and obstetric outcome in morbidly obese parturients, *Anesthesiology* 79 (1993): 1210–1218.
10. Perlow JH, Morgan MA. *American Journal of Obstetrics and Gynecology*, 560–565.
11. Perlow JH, Morgan MA, et al. *American Journal of Obstetrics and Gynecology*, 958–962.
12. Michlin R, Oettinger M, et al. *Journal of Perinatology*, 10–19.
13. Spellacy WN, et al. Macrosomia-maternal characteristics and infant complications, *Obstetrics and Gynecology* 66 (1985): 158.
14. Ramin SM, Cunningham F. Obesity in pregnancy, *Williams Obstetrics,* supplement, 19th ed. Appleton and Lange, June–July 1995.
15. *Ibid.*

Chapter 6

1. Martens MG, et al. Development of wound infection or separation after cesarean delivery: prospective evaluation of 2431 cases, *Journal of Reproductive Medicine* 40:3 (March 1995): 171–175.
2. Beattie PG, et al. Risk factors for wound infection following cesarean section, *Australian and New Zealand Journal of Obstetrics and Gynecology* 34:4 (Aug. 1994): 398–402.
3. Konje JC, et al. Pregnancy in obese women, *Journal of Obstetrics and Gynecology* 13 (1993): 413.
4. Naumann RW, et al. Subcutaneous tissue approximation in relation to

wound disruption after cesarean delivery in obese women, *Obstetrics and Gynecology* 85:3 (March 1995): 412–416.

5. Martens MG, et al. *Journal of Reproductive Medicine,* 171–175.
6. Isaccs J, et al. Obstetric challenges of massive obesity complicating pregnancy, *Journal of Perinatology* 14 (1994): 10–14.
7. Calandra C, et al. Maternal obesity in pregnancy, *Obstetrics and Gynecology* 57:1 (1981): 8–12.
8. Hood DD, Dewan DM. Anesthetic and obstetric outcome in morbidly obese parturients, *Anesthesiology* 79 (1993): 1210.

Chapter 9

1. *Manual of Clinical Dietetics,* 6th ed., American Dietetic Association, 2000, 121–122.
2. *Nutrition Action Newsletter* 8 (Sept. 2001). Center for Science in the Public Interest.

Chapter 11

1. *Kathy Smith's Pregnancy Workout,* produced by Kathy Smith Productions, Fox Hills Video, Media Home Entertainment Inc. (1989).
2. *Ibid.*
3. Exercise in Pregnancy. ACOG Technical Bulletin no. 189, *ACOG 2001 Compendium of Selected Publications* (Feb. 1994): 445–449.

Chapter 12

1. *Manual of Clinical Dietetics,* 6th ed., American Dietetic Association, 2000, 117.

INDEX

Page numbers in *italic* indicate illustrations; those in **bold** indicate charts and tables.